floating

feathers

*f*loating
*f*eathers

A DOCTOR'S
HARROWING EXPERIENCE
AS A PATIENT WITHIN
CONVENTIONAL MEDICINE

AND

AN IMPASSIONED CALL
FOR THE FUTURE OF CARE
IN AMERICA

Ross I.S. Zbar, MD

MILES
TREVOR
PRESS

Published by Miles Trevor Press
PO Box 252
Oakland, NJ 07436

For information about bulk orders, please contact the publisher at:
MilesTrevorPress@yahoo.com

ISBN: 978-1-7345416-0-1 pbk
ISBN: 978-1-7345416-1-8 hc
ISBN: 978-1-7345416-2-5 ebk

Library of Congress Control Number: 2020902278

Editing and book design by Stacey Aaronson

Printed in the United States of America

This book is dedicated to all those who have either helped or hindered my journey in life to this point, as it is the present that I gratefully embrace.

CONTENTS

author's note | i

TRAUMA

ROAD TO RECOVERY

ADVOCACY

author's note

Much of this book was composed only two months after my near-fatal accident while I was rehabilitating at home. The scars were still fresh and painful, but I was grateful to be capable of writing down my recollection of the events while they remained vivid. The descriptions in this book are my memories, as well as those of my wife and two stepchildren, who filled in the gaps that escaped me in the blackness of my trauma.

As a surgeon who dedicates his life to helping others, I never imagined that almost dying would make me a better physician, but it has. More importantly, this trauma has made me a better person. Best of all, as both physician and patient, I was given a unique opportunity to see how our system of medicine treats people, which sadly, in many ways, is replete with accepted protocols that are not only antiquated and injurious, but inhumane. It is my hope this book can be a catalyst to advance thoughtful dialogue of that system to make true positive change, one that will benefit medical personnel and patients alike.

Amor fati,
Ross I.S. Zbar, MD, FACS
Glen Ridge, NJ
October 2019

TRAUMA

chapter one

◆

December 22, 2018

It is an unusually warm Saturday afternoon in the Northeast, and I thankfully have the next few days off—no scheduled patients or surgeries because of the holidays. My two stepsons, Sotiri and Vasili, are home from college, and after finishing lunch with my wife and me, they excuse themselves and dash off to enjoy the break. I, too, get up from the table, poised to tackle my growing to-do list.

I spend my weekdays fixing holes in people as a plastic surgeon specializing in reconstruction, and I enjoy spending time on the weekends doing similar work on my house. In fact, I find that tending to "wounds" that don't bleed are much less stressful for me. Unlike in the operating room, I can eat and take breaks while tinkering as a handyman, and my house doesn't complain that the resulting scar is visible (although my wife may). On this particular day, first on the list is mending a new leak from a skylight in our bedroom.

I kiss my wife Denise and tell her how much I love her, then leave for the hardware store and purchase the items I need. After returning home, I take out the extension ladder and lean it against the roof. I climb up easily yet carefully, navigate to the skylight situated on a secondary roof, and inspect it. A small gap between the tar and metal frame is the culprit. I pull out the caulk gun and start to patch the hole, only to find that the caulking tube is nearly dried out and I need the spare one I've just purchased. My eldest stepson is on his way to the gym and offers to help, but I tell him I'm fine. We chat for a few minutes, me on the roof and him on the pavers. Then he drives off.

The next thing I know, I am encased in a padded hive of drones and beeps. My vision is blurry; people slide past like abstract brushstrokes. It takes only a few moments to realize that I'm in an intensive-care unit. Through what feels like a rainy fog, my wife leans close to my face and softly tells me that I fell and suffered major injuries. At first, I don't believe her. Then she tells me that I've been here for three weeks, that I've missed Christmas and New Year's. *That's impossible*, I think. But then, slowly, warbled memories begin to play in my mind. Bizarre hallucinations. Misty snapshots of my wife talking to me. Severe discomfort. A strong sense of being imprisoned.

I also vividly recall being haunted by a deep feeling of dread that I was, for days on end, fighting against the Angel of Death.

chapter two

I come from a family of physicians and medical practitioners: my paternal grandfather, who emigrated from Poland,
and my father practiced otolaryngology (a focus on ears, nose,
and throat, also known as ENT); my maternal grandfather was
an internist in the Village of New York City; and my mother
was a nurse. I clearly remember being a high school student,
sitting in a study carrel, knowing I would walk the same path
of medicine my family had—only I wanted to be a plastic surgeon. As an Eagle Scout, I was inculcated with giving back to
others, and I was always attracted to the idea of performing
cleft-lip surgery in developing countries.

I worked hard in school in pursuit of my dream and was
privileged to attend Harvard College and Yale Medical School,
followed by a surgical internship at Lenox Hill Hospital in New
York City, then a residency in otolaryngology at the University
of Iowa.

At the time, Iowa was ranked as the most competitive
ENT program nationally, but my east-coast friends and family
couldn't fathom my moving there. It was a big leap for me too,
but I was filled with ambition the day I shipped off from New
York to Iowa City, driving directly west for a thousand miles.
My younger brother, Brett, rode shotgun to help me navigate
the urban sprawl of the country's most congested region to the

endless cornfields of the Midwest. I had never smelled hog farms until that drive.

During the four years I lived in Iowa City, I learned the true meaning of "Midwestern values"—an honest day's work for an honest day's pay, modesty matters, your word is your bond, and your name and reputation is your most prized possession—all qualities I valued as well. Perhaps it is because so many Iowans grew up in farming that my Ivy League education was no match for the sincere humility and sensibility that Midwesterners possess.

Being at the University of Iowa also afforded me a rare opportunity to work in a laboratory that was studying genetic deafness, and I leapt at the chance to participate. I would spend two three-month stints performing medical research in rural southern India, where there is a high rate of consanguineous marriage. Because of this, I was able to draw blood and extract DNA from members of the same family, helping to isolate genes causing deafness. It was my time in India that solidified my desire to perform surgeries in the developing world.

To become a plastic surgeon during the 1990s, one had to be board certified in another surgical specialty, so choosing otolaryngology seemed natural to me. During one of my ENT rotations in Des Moines, I applied to the University of Texas Southwestern Medical Center's Department of Plastic Surgery —arguably the best in the country—and was accepted. So, after finishing my first residency in Iowa City, I moved to Dallas. Once again, Brett helped me make the drive—one he'll never let me forget. I had loaded the U-Haul trailer with all my heavy books in the back, figuring those were the least important items. As a result, we fishtailed the entire eight-hundred-mile drive; we couldn't drive more than forty-five miles an hour without risking a turnover. The trip took forever, but it turned out to be an eye-opening adventure, from the plains of Iowa to the oil rigs of Oklahoma on to Big D.

After settling in at Parkland Hospital for my training in plastic surgery, I was stealing a break on a particularly rough on-call night and noted a flier in the hallway. An organization called Interplast was offering a first-time fellowship for a recent graduate to spend an entire year traveling the globe while performing and teaching cleft surgery. This was cosmic alignment. The fellowship was sponsored by the granddaughter of Jerome Webster, MD, a famous plastic surgeon who not only started the division at Columbia University but traveled the world lecturing and elevating the standard of care.

I earned an interview for the position, which was held in a luxurious New York City hotel. I had just plowed through Thomas Wolfe's *A Man in Full*, and I found myself channeling the protagonist during my interview. His belief was that when presented with an opportunity, any opportunity, a person's action—or inaction—reflects his or her true character. This fellowship was an opportunity to prove my commitment to helping people. I even went so far as to criticize the interview venue as being hypocritical, given the position they were looking to fill. Afterward, I realized that expressing myself so candidly was probably a mistake, and I figured I had blown it. But it turned out that one of the interviewers, unbeknownst to me, was the medical director of Interplast at the time—David Dingman, MD—and a huge Ayn Rand fan. He identified with my speech about principles. He had even named one of his daughters after the female lead of *Atlas Shrugged*: Dagny. He compared my interview to John Galt's soliloquy about the power of individualism, and it was clear we were in complete agreement with the belief that a person's daily actions should reflect his or her moral principles.

I ended up getting the fellowship and was thrilled to learn he would direct it. David was the son of a world-famous plastic surgeon, Reed Dingman, MD, who is still considered a giant in our specialty. I was also delighted to find out that David was not only an adventurous soul like me but ascribed to the ancient Marcus Aurelius quote from *Meditations* that I loved: "Stop talking about what the good man is like, and just be one." David served as my professional mentor and friend while we worked at Interplast. He's the one who taught me about the black-and-white moral issues of life—but how the grays were the ones that were so hard to navigate.

AFTER TWO YEARS of training in plastic surgery, I completed my residency and started my one-year overseas fellowship, traveling the world with multiple teams performing cleft surgery in developing countries. Because this was two years before the 9-11 World Trade Center attacks of 2001, it was a different time. I had no concerns flying internationally to work side by side with local plastic surgeons in Nepal, India, Sri Lanka, Peru, Ecuador, Cambodia, and Vietnam. In fact, I relished it.

It was during this time at Interplast that one of the volunteer American plastic surgeons gave me a sage piece of advice: to continue living like a resident once I started my private practice. I knew what he meant. Too many doctors become arrogant and caught up in their presumed power; over time they forget why they went into medicine, becoming too embroiled in hospital politics, and trading quality patient care for a misguided focus on making money. He not only suggested I save money whenever I could and not spend my income frivolously, he also encouraged me to continue to pursue my academic goals.

I took that advice to heart.

After I completed my fellowship in August of 2000, I returned to my hometown in northern New Jersey and opened my private practice. I had found the Interplast volunteer work so rewarding that I continued leading cleft trips for several years afterward, eventually joining another volunteer surgery group —Iowa MOST (Miles of Smiles Team), medically directed by a fellow Iowa ENT graduate and mentor of mine who is also a plastic surgeon, John Canady, MD. That group concentrated mainly on patients in Guatemala. I loved taking care of patients in my private practice and volunteering abroad, while also performing frequent cleft-lip surgeries at a local charity hospital that focused on the poor.

I never imagined that almost twenty years later, that same charity hospital would be responsible for saving my life.

chapter three

◆

DENISE

December 22, 2018

I am still in my pajamas, doing housework in preparation for Ross's parents' arrival tomorrow for the holidays. I heard Ross's car return from the hardware store a while ago, but not much of a sound since, so I peek out through the side door window to check on him. In front of the garage, I see the ladder lying flat, with Ross's twisted body next to it. I immediately think he's playing a joke on us—he knows Vasili is playing Fortnite with his headphones on, and that he has an unobstructed view to the driveway. Since Ross is always kidding around with me, I'm certain he's trying to frighten one or both of us. He frequently plays hoaxes like this, as he is obsessed with preparing me for when he dies; as a surgeon, he knows how fragile life is and how quickly it ends, so he often does things like drill me on his computer passwords, or quiz me on where documents are kept in the event he is incapacitated. He's even faked his death by kissing me good night and falling on top of me, making me push his dead weight off.

Today seems no different. I truly believe this is yet another test and that he will stand up and give a good laugh that he fooled me, so I open the side door and play along.

"Ross, you okay?" I call out.

He starts to moan, asking what happened.

Normally, I would roll my eyes, but something about his voice seems off. I sprint over to him and find a large pool of blood by his head. He lifts his head slightly and attempts to get up.

"I can't feel my legs," he says.

I immediately know he's not playing some elaborate prank as my heart drops. "Vasili!" I scream. I run into the house, grab the cordless phone, and dial 911. I dash back outside as the dispatcher's gentle voice tells me to remain calm and stay with Ross until the paramedics arrive. "Keep him engaged in conversation," she says. "Make sure he doesn't move in the event there's a spinal injury." She stays with me on the phone for minutes that feel like hours until someone arrives.

The police reach the house first, rushing toward Ross with a defibrillator. The local ambulance squad is next, followed by the paramedics. They quickly take over, and I steal the opportunity to run upstairs to change out of my pajamas. I throw on the closest jeans and sweater and grab my purse. I run back downstairs to see my husband still lying on the driveway with even more blood pooling around him.

Vasili has called his brother, and Sotiri has sped back from the gym. Vasili tells me the police have inspected the area to make sure it was an accident and not attempted murder. That thought never even crossed my mind. The next thing I know, the paramedics are strapping Ross onto a backboard. They had cut open his clothes with trauma shears to inspect his injuries, and as they move him, feathers from his favorite down vest gently drift into the air, following him into the ambulance.

"We need to take him to a trauma center," the ambulance driver barks, snapping me away from the surreal scene that's moving as if in slow motion. "You can sit in the front with me. You're not allowed in the back."

I nod and climb into the passenger seat as the paramedics continue working on Ross. I call his parents several times. No answer. I text EMERGENCY and call again. They finally pick up.

"It's serious," I tell them frantically, giving the details I know.

"Was he alert when you found him?" my father-in-law asks.

"Yes," I confirm.

"We'll leave right away and meet you at the hospital," he says. They are forty-five minutes away.

I inform the driver that I work at one of the campuses of a large hospital system and insist that we go to their trauma center.

She smiles politely. "We actually recommend going to a different trauma center."

When I start to protest, the young paramedic in the back empathetically chimes in. "If Ross were my father, I'd want him transported to this one. They're better equipped to deal with this kind of trauma because they see major injuries all the time."

I realize then how naive I am, how unaware of the severity of Ross's accident, as I watch them start an intravenous line of fentanyl and propofol. I am shocked by the fentanyl—I know it is a street drug used by addicts. But in this case, it is for Ross's benefit, to ease his pain and awareness.

The ambulance ride is dreadfully slow. The driver purposely takes it easy to minimize bumps and takes side roads to avoid traffic on the main route. Ross is in so much pain that they increase the dose of fentanyl.

"I know there was a lot of blood," the driver says, trying to reassure me. My body is twisted so that my eyes are glued to my husband. "He'll be okay," she insists.

But it is a futile effort to calm me down. I finally turn and look out the window. *If only we went out to lunch . . . if only we decided to spend the day hiking . . . if only it were colder outside to have kept him inside . . . if only . . . if only.*

WHEN WE FINALLY arrive at the hospital, the trauma team is waiting for us. They whisk Ross off and instruct me to wait in one of the emergency bays.

I drift into an empty one, wanting privacy. I close the curtains so the staff can't see me and allow my welling emotion to take over. I am purposely quiet at first so no one can hear me, but my tears quickly evolve into sobs as complete devastation sets in. I fall to the floor and let it all flow out, in disbelief of how our lives have permanently changed in an instant.

Suddenly, I hear my name. "Yes?" I manage.

Someone eases the curtain back a little. It's the ambulance driver. "Here are his things," she says gently, handing me Ross's ripped clothes and a bag containing his watch, belt, and cell phone. His wallet is missing, and I feel awkward asking about it, so I don't.

"Thank you," I mutter, and she disappears.

Shortly afterward, Vasili and Sotiri arrive at the hospital. They stayed behind to put the ladder away and move Ross's car into the garage, then they cleaned Ross's blood off the driveway. They didn't want their stepdad upset seeing pavers stained with his blood. They also know I'm barely holding on and that I couldn't see the blood without experiencing a complete breakdown.

As I impatiently wait in the bay with the boys, hoping for

any positive information, the trauma doctor steps in and casually explains that Ross is now going for CT scans and X-rays.

"I'll be back with updates as they're available," he assures me.

One of the nurses tells me that the medical director of the trauma service did two tours of duty in Afghanistan with the US Army, which alleviates my concerns about the staff having ample experience. In fact, I'm grateful that this team is looking after Ross. As promised, the on-call chief comes out of the trauma slot with updates every few minutes. But each time, he informs us of a new injury on a different body part; the severity of the trauma is more and more magnified. Ross has ten rib fractures on the left; a clavicle and scapula fracture on the same side; three rib fractures on the right; a sacral fracture; and a massive hematoma on his left thigh and buttock. He also has a temporal bone fracture on the left with paralysis on the left side of his face. Most devastatingly, he has two intraparenchymal (between the functional tissue in the brain) hemorrhagic contusions in the right temporal lobe and one in the right inferior frontal lobe. Shockingly to all of us, with his myriad injuries, Ross still has all his teeth.

When Ross's parents arrive from Manhattan, the doctors give them a full update. Being in the medical world, they know what Ross is facing. Sotiri feels for them, and in his thoughtfulness calls Ross's brother, who is away with his family on vacation in France, to let him know what has happened.

When my father-in-law finds out, he scolds, "Why did you do that? You shouldn't have disturbed Brett's vacation when there's nothing they can do."

I glance sympathetically at Sotiri, at a loss to understand that logic. It is precisely at times like these that you need the love and support of family, not an added level of tension.

We sit in awkward silence for a bit until we are told that all five of us can go into the trauma room together. We witness the well-coordinated trauma team in action as they continue to work on Ross. Shortly afterward, we're told his blood count is very low, which is why he's receiving multiple transfusions.

"He's still actively bleeding in his leg," one of the team says.

Within seconds, Ross is transferred to interventional radiology where they perform a procedure on torn arteries with coils. In my state of anguish, I am happy to discover that the radiologist performing the procedure works with Ross at the same hospital where he attends. Though I'm reassured by this connection, I'm worried to learn that Ross keeps removing his supplemental oxygen.

"Maybe you can help," the radiologist says.

I follow him into the procedure room. With Ross losing so much blood, compounded by his severe injuries, it's not easy to get him to cooperate, and it's clear he's somewhat confused.

"Take this fucking thing off me," Ross growls. "I'm fine."

I'm a little embarrassed, but his noncompliant attitude gives me hope that perhaps he might make it through.

AFTER THE COIL procedure, Ross is transported to the surgical intensive care unit (SICU) and they assure me that he is stable.

"But," the doctors warn, "he may need to be intubated. He'll probably have trouble breathing because of the multiple rib fractures. Outside of his brain injury, Ross's breathing will be the main issue that needs management."

We sit vigil for hours, but after sunset we are told that visitors aren't allowed to remain in the SICU during the night. Although I can't imagine leaving Ross alone, I reluctantly agree to return in the morning—or sooner if need be.

The boys and I arrive back home, grateful that the darkness obscures the scene of Ross's accident. We wearily say goodnight to each other and retire to our rooms. As I look around in a daze, Ross's absence is palpable. I catch sight of his wallet on the nightstand and feel a momentary sense of relief. But the empty bed brings me to tears once again and I fall onto it, crying myself into a fitful sleep.

In the middle of the night, my cell phone rings. I bolt awake and grab it quickly. The number on my screen is the hospital. My heart accelerates as I answer, knowing the news can't be good.

A physician sympathetically informs me that Ross was unable to breathe and had to be intubated. Though I'm hopeful it is merely a temporary situation, I fear deep down that our lives from here on out will never be the same.

THE FOLLOWING MORNING, the sun wakes me through the skylight and reality rushes in like a knife to my heart. When I drag myself out of bed and down the stairs, I am relieved when I look out the window that the boys scrubbed the blood off the driveway. But I am startled to see something else: in the daylight, tiny fragments seem to hover over our driveway. For a moment, I'm confused. But when I look closer, I realize they are feathers—errant feathers from Ross's vest still floating eerily as if he had just been spirited away.

chapter four

I became a physician because helping people has always been important to me. But I am also an iconoclast in that I subscribe to the two-thousand-year-old Latin expression, "*Quis custodiet ipsos custodes*," which translates as, "Who watches the watchmen?" In other words, we must always hold the powerful to account.

Throughout my life, I've found myself disagreeing with various individuals because of this passion for questioning the validity of authority. It's never been uncommon for me, when appropriate, to question hospital administrators with regard to our Hippocratic mission: giving outstanding patient care. I have even debated my residency mentors at times when they seem to drift away from patient-driven healthcare. I wholeheartedly believe we must always treat patients as we would our own families. This sometimes bucks the system and ruffles feathers, but it is critical we not lose sight of our primary goal. It's true that persistently delivering phenomenal patient care requires a commitment that is challenging in the real world, but to me that is no excuse. We, as healthcare providers, are given a remarkable gift to help people in a significant way, and I could never allow myself to compromise. The bottom line is: we must never forget that our patients need us, no matter the cost.

During my years in this profession, I've tragically witnessed medicine metamorphose. It's no secret that it has been taken over by corporations and that many healthcare workers feel powerless. How can physicians successfully advocate for their patients if they are employed by a financial conglomerate? How can nurses speak up about patient safety if they are paid by a hospital focused on financially driven metrics? Private equity backs a large part of today's medical care, and, as a result, profit is now frequently placed above patients. This means that seemingly minor but critical decisions, such as referrals for treatment, are not always in the best interest of the patient.

The United States has arguably the greatest healthcare system in the world, but most (not all) facilities focus on the wrong objective. Sadly, in the current marketplace, increasing patient volume for the sake of profit is now what drives healthcare. Although medical care in most of the US is adequate, it is not as phenomenal as it could be, which is not only tragic but a crime. To date, the solutions presented in Washington DC are of little help. Metrics in medicine focus on supposed quality indicators, which, for those of us in the trenches, is of laughable and questionable merit. For one, the entire electronic medical record (EMR) system serves as a giant cash register, with healthcare workers shackled to it instead of performing more needed direct patient care. I am not alone in my beliefs, but few healthcare professionals verbalize their concerns about the commercialization of healthcare for fear of becoming pariahs.

Many industry leaders claim it is burnout that fuels this epidemic of frustrated and demoralized healthcare workers. But there is a significant problem using the term "burnout" as applied to physicians. The term is, in fact, a form of victim shaming because it implies those who experience it fail to be strong. The term furthermore suggests that those who have burnout are not resilient. This could not be further from the truth. How can people who survive years of tortuous education, from college to post-graduate training, supposedly not be strong enough in the current environment? These same industry leaders additionally say that it is burnout that leads to disruptive behavior by physicians. Rather, as many people are realizing, a more accurate term for what physicians—and all healthcare workers for that matter—are currently experiencing is moral insult, or even moral injury. In other words, they are enduring trauma from being forced to face tasks that transgress their moral beliefs. Dr. Lissa Rankin has further posited that the torturous, sleep-deprived regimen physicians experience—from medical school on—is actually no different from what the military experiences on a battlefield, resulting in a pure form of post-traumatic stress disorder (PTSD). When you combine the two, it's no wonder that physician suicide is at an all-time high.

Witnessing overworked, understaffed nurses waste time focused on entering meaningless data into the computer in order to capture and maximize charges, instead of carefully reading my thoughtfully crafted paperwork that explains the patient's medical situation, brings me great personal pain. These daily chores geared to benefit the corporation are not why people dedicate their lives to healthcare.

When I find out one of my patients has suffered a needless complication, like a fall out of bed, due to cost-cutting measures of the facility, there are two victims as a result: not only is my patient physically hurt from the fall, but I am hurt too, in the moral sense. When my colleagues remain silent, fearing that whistleblowing will lead to their own destruction, we have further cause of creating a second victim.

Before my accident, I was personally struggling with these major philosophical issues. One of the local hospitals in which I am an attending physician had been sold to a new company (based in a different time zone). I ran for vice president of the medical staff with the sole intention of spearheading correction of numerous patient safety lapses, exacerbated by financial decisions made by the administration in its zealous and arguably insane profiteering. In my campaign for the position, I made it clear that patient safety was my primary focus, and I won the election by an overwhelming majority of the medical staff vote.

This position of vice president was designed to transition to the presidency after two years of service. Arguably, I was an idiot. A big idiot. Although I had published numerous manuscripts in peer-reviewed literature on the career dangers physicians face when whistleblowing, I nevertheless drove myself—electively—into this self-destructive process. These papers were co-authored with industry leaders and attorneys—one of which, from nearly a decade prior, had been cited numerous times in both US and Canadian scientific literature. This study (known as the "pariah" paper) described in stifling detail how the controlling powers in a hospital can inappropriately flag and consequently derail a physician who is championing patient safety by labeling him or her as disruptive. (The moniker "disruptive" not only applies to a physician on staff who is emotionally or physically abusive to other healthcare workers by treating them without respect, but bizarrely can be tagged to a physician who interferes with the economic/financial goals of the hospital.) This strategic maneuver essentially wrecks the physician while protecting the hospital from negative exposure. The paper went on to conclude, perhaps naively, how a physician champion should work within the system to change it.

In summary, I thought I could live my scientific conclusions, but instead it was the classic setup for failure. In my case, some recent events at this facility put the patients at such grave risk that I was incapable of remaining silent. Inaction was equivalent to tacit approval. The final straw in this epic battle occurred shortly thereafter. Without getting too technical, the contracts of the hospital mandated that professional medical services—such as radiology, anesthesiology, pathology, or emergency-room care—remain in-network with the same insurance programs with which the hospital participated. These are services in-patients may have no choice but to utilize, and I was aware of this policy from the time I served on the board of trustees. These rules guaranteed that patients weren't hit with surprise bills by services rendered in the hospital.

During this time, many of the employed physicians in some of the above-mentioned fields were forced to join a company that was run by an individual who was closely collaborating with the hospital administration. Suddenly, a number of my patients were noting out-of-network balance billing. When I brought this up with the administration of the hospital, I was told it was simply a billing error. But I wasn't convinced. Multiple patients were receiving these bills, and a well-respected surgical colleague of mine reported the same for his patients. Denise and I had even received one for our eldest son who required a surgery. So did another physician on staff when she, too, had surgery. Furthermore, one of my colleagues, employed by this very same entity, reported that he was indeed out-of-network for several insurance plans. I went online and verified this to be true. As a patient advocate, I had made the "mistake" of caring too much—and there was no way I was going to turn my head now that it was clear to me financial games were being played and that money was trumping morality.

I wrote a well-crafted and very polite email to those in charge, asking that we investigate the practice. The response?

All hell broke loose. I was told I was being disruptive to the mission of the hospital—and I was sidelined by the corporation's chief medical officer, who asked that I consider voluntarily attending a course on communications so that moving forward, I would learn "not to offend people." I knew this type of bullying frequently occurred in the corporate world—employees must support their corporation—but I was not an employee. I am engaged by patients in a doctor-patient relationship to not only improve their health but represent and help guide them through the Byzantine process of our country's healthcare system. This is precisely the type of moral conflict in which physicians find themselves daily. And because this type of corruption is a significant driving force behind healthcare, most of us feel no choice but to remain silent. Bottom line: The corporatization of healthcare has resulted in the loss of morality.

FOR THE NEXT year, I maintained a low profile so that I could evolve unchallenged into the presidency of the medical staff and have a shot at changing the world. But the administration didn't want me to become president of the medical staff; they already thought of me as a "disruptor" to the financial bottom line and feared I would shine a light on the areas of patient care that needed improvement. Clearly, the best person to enumerate considerations in patient safety and care at a facility is an independent practitioner with a medical or nursing degree, not a hired individual who is focused principally on profit. Yet, the opposite is precisely what happens when money rules and is worshipped like a god. Executive teams are driven to protect their interests at all costs when the one true goal is to make the corporation more money.

So, to maintain my trajectory—despite the odds against me—I tried to work within the system by writing polite emails, refraining from engaging people directly to improve failing quality, and filing electronic reports documenting gaps in quality. In so doing, I was striving to exemplify the very conclusions I reached in my "pariah" manuscript from the previous decade. Of course, physicians were repeatedly told that in any highly reliable organization, quality reports would be taken seriously and there would never be the risk of retaliation for whistleblowing. But once I took it to the next level and started frequently filing these quality reports that objectively documented patient endangerment, I became an easy and justifiable target for the administration, which remained focused on profit.

After bringing these lapses in patient safety to light via the reporting system, I received a letter signed by the corporation's chief medical officer (CMO) and a local doctor who personally benefited from significant financial entanglements with this facility. It was now evident to me that I had a massive bullseye on my back. The letter, clearly demonstrating crony capitalism at its finest, unfairly accused me of bullying behavior. This jury of two was stacked with individuals paid directly by the same corporation where I was trying to correct policies that were undeniably harming patients—and they were fighting me even though I had been duly elected by the medical staff. The accusations made against me were baseless: the CMO stated that he performed an "investigation," but when I asked multiple times to provide examples, he never revealed to me specific details of a single event he found concerning. Even the local doctor who signed the letter sheepishly admitted to me in a subsequent phone conversation that he was never made aware of any specific events. When I asked why he signed the false letter, he didn't answer. I never had an opportunity to face my accusers; in fact, I was sure there were *no* accusers, only people solicited by the corporation. These people were likely asked something ridiculous about me, such as did I ever look at them in a way they didn't like.

Bottom line: I never stood a chance.

You can imagine the dichotomy in which I was trapped. On the one hand, I was told I should deal directly with staff who weren't meeting quality standards, not their supervisors; on the other, I was told I shouldn't discuss issues directly with staff as they found it threatening. The worst part was that as this was happening, patients were suffering unnecessarily.

Essentially, I was being forced to remain silent. But how can a physician stay quiet when employee errors can cause harm? I couldn't.

In the well-crafted words of Mark Twain:

"Whenever you find yourself on the side of the majority, it is time to pause and reflect."

In the view of the corporation, my attempt to politely but persistently decrease the patient fall rate, improve the electronic medical records system, identify delinquent nursing, and educate the operating room staff in proper surgical technique was inappropriate. None of my actions, they insisted, were fitting for a member of the medical staff leadership to champion in the hospital. Ironically, I could not turn to the board of trustees for a fair investigation, as a close friend of the CEO was president—a doctor employed by the very same corporation he was supposedly overseeing. Interestingly, the previous president of the board had been an intelligent and dedicated private citizen, who also happened to be an attorney. I wasn't surprised to learn that he was quickly outmaneuvered by the corporation and that he smartly resigned when he realized there was no hope of slaying the beast. The fact that this behavior was permitted was unbelievable.

I want to be clear that all of this subterfuge did nothing to raise the hospital's quality ranking. In fact, it rendered the opposite. The hospital repeatedly earned Cs—which would plummet to a D—from the reputable Leapfrog Hospital Surveys that provide objective evidence of significantly poor quality. I, of course, had seen this coming and tried to help patients avoid unnecessary risk. But instead of viewing my efforts as positive for the hospital and its patients, the administration saw my concern as a barrier to earning more money, not an opportunity to address significant gaps in patient care. In short, it was easier to eliminate me rather than address the major quality issues.

This was when I made one of the hardest decisions in my career. In this David versus Goliath battle, I was an underdog. I knew I couldn't hope to triumph; the corporation had much deeper pockets than mine, and one cannot win when fighting cheaters. I therefore resigned as vice president (and potential future president) of the medical staff and took my surgical volume out of that hospital, vowing to bring patients only to facilities that repeatedly earned high marks from Leapfrog.

As you can imagine, this was a devastating event in my life. I realized, without a shadow of a doubt, three highly disturbing facts: 1) that the corporatization of healthcare means that people who fight for patients are viewed as blocking the real goal of the owners and investors: profits; 2) that there is no true oversight from an objective governing body; and 3) that the executives at these profit-hungry facilities treat doctors who champion quality care simply as obstacles to be overrun.

And then I became a patient.

chapter five

◆

ROSS
ICU Delirium

I am restless but can't move much. My body is screaming all over. I feel trapped and can't escape . . . why am I tied down? What have I done to be imprisoned? I'm being grilled about something I didn't do . . . I'm innocent but no one believes me . . .

⬭

I have to perform a challenging major surgical procedure in under an hour. I need to finish quickly so I can go home to my family. I'm working as fast as I can but something's wrong. Something's not working. I have to start over. I don't have enough time. I can't get home until I finish, but I don't have the right surgical instruments. The patient needs help, and I need to finish so I can go home, but nothing I'm doing is working the way it's supposed to . . .

⬭

I have a terribly sick patient. I try and try to make her better but nothing works. My heart is racing. "Somebody help!" Doctors and nurses stand around me but they just stare, doing nothing . . .

◇

I'm trying to get home. I'm being held prisoner. It looks like a hospital but is in the head of the Statue of Liberty. People are hunched over desks, scanning computers as if they are in a control tower. Picturesque windows overlook New York Harbor. My goal is to locate a young child in the city and save him. I am crying. I can't get out of my cell and I pound on the wall. "This is unfair! I can't get out!" I glance around panicked, but nobody looks at me. I pound, and pound, and pound . . .

◇

I've lived through a similar trauma in the past. I believe it with complete certainty. I was recently hospitalized for tracheal stenosis and forgot to tell my family. This type of breathing problem happened to me before. I blurt out the name of a surgeon who performed a procedure on me in Philadelphia. Denise asks my father if this is true.

"No," he says definitively.

Why is he lying? Why doesn't anyone believe me?

◇

I hear music. They are familiar songs. These are the ones I listen to in the OR while I'm working. It is amazing. I can perform surgeries I never performed before . . .

◇

A song from high school is playing . . . it is by Kate Bush. Certain lyrics play over and over:

    And if I only could
    I'd make a deal with God
    And I'd get him to swap our places . . .

◇

It is evening. I'm tired from our long day.
    "Can we go back to our hotel room?" I ask Denise.
She looks sad.
    "Aren't we on vacation?" I ask.
She slowly shakes her head . . .

◇

I am severely constipated. An enormous bowel movement is stuck in my rectum. I know I must use my fingers to dislodge it. I reach in and pull it out, but it is attached to a string. I pull on the string but it won't end. It just keeps coming and coming . . .

◇

"Do you know who I am?" my wife's beautiful face asks, framed by angelic clouds. I feel her positive energy flow through me. I see her hand reaching from the sky to pick me up . . .

◇

I am trapped in the seatbelt of the driver's seat, dangling up-side down. There was an accident. My car flipped and a foot-ball flew from the dashboard and lodged in my throat. I open my mouth and reach down into it. I grab the football and pull it out. I have to do it to stay alive . . .

◆

chapter six

DENISE

Day Two and Forever

My new reality is the fear of phone calls of tragic status updates in the middle of the night, or worse, that Ross didn't make it. And the feathers . . . the feathers appear everywhere. Floating over our driveway. Lodged in the cobwebs of our garage. Nestled in the landscaping. They seem to represent the ongoing fragility of life, mocking our ignorant belief that we can control things. Change is the only constant. And we should be grateful for positive changes, but how do I shift my perception to a positive one when I think of the change that's occurred in our lives? How can it possibly be a good thing that my husband is fighting for his life?

I SIT AT Ross's bedside from 8:00 a.m. to 9:00 p.m. every day. I've taken family leave and put my life on hold. I'm convinced that if Ross is going to make it through this ordeal, he needs to be guarded. Although the doctors and nurses strive to be conscientious, errors do happen, and I don't want my husband suffering from one of them if I can help it.

I've done my best to make sure my boys have a decent Christmas break from school, but there isn't much I can do. It's also frustrating that Ross's parents come and go, merely fitting him into their schedule, whereas Ross *is* my schedule. They frequently ask if I want to join them for dinner at a local restaurant, and all I can think is, *How can you go out to dinner when your son is lying on what could be his deathbed? How is it humanly possible to be so detached from your own child?*

When Ross's brother returns from his vacation in France, a week after the injury, he exhibits the same coldness. After only a brief stay at the hospital on Saturday morning, he tells me he's leaving to meet his parents for lunch a few towns away. It is then that I wonder if Ross's father and brother with their medical degrees are simply too scientific in their manner to offer love-based emotional support. It is untenable to me, but that's what they project. For me, now is the time to witness Ross's critical journey and pray for his recovery, not merely ask medical-related questions and leave after getting the answers.

It is abundantly clear to me that they may be his family, but they don't know my husband. I'm at his bedside thirteen hours a day, and I see him move all of his limbs and communicate the best way he can on a daily basis. I know for certain that this is not the time to give up on the man I love with all my heart.

FOR THE NEXT week, Ross remains intubated. His massive left leg hematoma consolidates, resulting in acute swelling of his testicles, which are now purple in color and distended beyond belief. The compassionate nurses assure me that this is not dangerous, but I am terrified of what might happen. For now, that is the only alarming distension we can see. But I am told that if his brain swells, the surgeons may need to remove part of his skull to relieve pressure. For days I am on pins and needles, but thankfully, this surgery is not required.

At a certain point, the trauma team decides to test if Ross

can breathe on his own. They carefully remove the endotracheal tube, which is a huge relief for Ross, but his mouth is so dry that he's unable to talk. Despite his discomfort, he gives monumental effort to breathing, but with his multiple rib fractures, he's simply in too much pain and they must reinsert the breathing tube.

Witnessing my husband's struggle creates an unimaginable weight on my heart. My mother shares my anguish when she arrives and sees Ross intubated and sedated. It is oddly comforting when she breaks down with me at his ICU bedside.

THE NEXT DAY, Sunday (day eight)—in the midst of the two full days it's taking me to fill out the paperwork to become Ross's power of attorney—the trauma team becomes concerned about the extent of the rib damage impeding Ross's ability to breathe on his own and orders a three-dimensional CT reconstruction of his chest. Ross's parents and brother are with me when the chief of trauma shows us the scans of Ross's ribs broken in multiple places with shards sticking out. I can only imagine how painful it is for my husband to simply breathe. The damage appears so extensive that we fear Ross may never get off the ventilator.

"I suggest a surgery called rib plating," the Army veteran doctor says.

He explains the procedure in detail, describing that his goal is to plate as many ribs as possible to stabilize—or "fixate"—the chest wall, which will help Ross breathe on his own. It is a relatively new procedure and there is not much data available. The truth is, not many people survive these types of injuries to become a candidate for the fixation procedure.

"Here," he says, "I'll show you how it works." He draws pictures of how the hardware can stabilize the ribs, keeping them together so they can heal faster. "I believe this plating will give Ross a greater chance of getting off the ventilator. It should decrease the pain and allow for better chest wall movement." He also suggests that the orthopedic surgeon can fix Ross's broken clavicle at the same time to expedite healing and rehabilitation.

A FEW HOURS later, the surgical team comes to get my consent. They tell me that the trauma team is set to perform the rib plating, but they cannot promise that the orthopedic surgeon will be available to fix the clavicle.

"Why should my husband be subjected to a separate surgery just because of a scheduling issue?" I assert. "If I have to call the chief of orthopedics, I will. If he's not available, I'll work my way down the staff roster of orthopedic surgeons until I find someone who is."

At that, the trauma team assures me that they'll locate an orthopedic surgeon who will make him or herself available for the procedure.

THE FOLLOWING DAY, on New Year's Eve, the surgery takes place. It requires six hours to plate the ribs, and Ross suffers a pneumothorax (collapsed lung) during the procedure. The surgeons attribute this to his positioning. When they perform a bronchoscopy to inspect the lung for damage, they determine Ross requires chest tubes on each side. After those are inserted, the orthopedic surgeon repairs the clavicle, which takes an additional three hours.

When Ross is returned to the ICU, he is placed in a bay next to a patient on contact precautions. This means the patient carries an easily transmissible pathogen that could cause major infection in compromised individuals. In Ross's weakened state, he could easily catch a resistant bacterium if a healthcare worker inadvertently forgets to wash his or her hands. I'm well aware that handwashing has been proven to decrease infections, but in some facilities it is poorly enforced.

"I need my husband moved," I insist to one of the nurses.

It takes some firm negotiating, but Ross is moved to a different slot. I know that one of his gravest risks is a hospital-acquired complication; an infection or a blood clot stands a better chance of killing Ross at this point than his actual fall, and there is no way I can let that happen to him. It would not only destroy me, but it would be a cruel joke on him after spending so much of his career working with hospitals to improve their safety.

ROSS IS SEDATED for several days to keep him comfortable, as no one in the ICU can figure out how to manage the new pain pump they embedded in Ross during the rib surgery. I am slightly frustrated but it doesn't get resolved, so I'm left to accept his sedation.

Soon after, Ross develops a fever. They diagnose pneumonia and start him on antibiotics, removing all but one of the chest tubes. Time seems to crawl as one malady after another slowly strangles my soulmate.

ANGER HAS BECOME an unwanted, but constant, companion when I'm alone. While driving to the hospital, or pulling into the garage at night, I scream at the top of my lungs. It's all I can do to break the overwhelming quiet.

I am furious at God. *Why did you let Ross fall?* I demand. As if God doesn't know my husband, I feel the need to supply reasons he deserves better than he's gotten. *He's such a good person. He spends so much time helping destitute patients over-*

seas. He's the most loving husband and stepfather. In my mind, it's truly as if none of that matters to the entity who's supposed to love us all unconditionally.

I am angry at our house—so much so that I'm ready to put it up for sale. How could it betray Ross this way? Every moment at home is a reminder that it "allowed" him to fall. The new dent in the gutter is proof that Ross tried to hang on but the house wouldn't let him.

And I'm mad at myself. If I had kept my mouth shut about the skylight leak after the rain that morning, Ross never would have climbed up on the roof.

This anger is the undercurrent of my accompanying pain and fear.

I haven't been able to look at Ross's clothes in our shared walk-in closet without crying; the suit he wore to work the day before his fall is sitting on the stool, not yet hung; the dry cleaning he picked up the morning of his trauma hangs on a hook. Eventually, I summon the strength to put all his clothes away, carefully folding them, not knowing if he'll ever wear them again. If he does, I wonder, *Will I need to help him get dressed every morning?*

I move the Christmas gifts, unopened, into the attic and discard the Christmas tree early.

I cannot even look at Ross's lunchbox, the childlike *Star Trek*–themed one he bought on the Internet that he brings daily to work. He uses it as a joke, but also as a way of showing people he doesn't follow normal convention. "It's a Stoic exercise to experience embarrassment on purpose to prove to oneself the world continues," he told me, supporting his iconoclastic behavior. "The judgments of other people are meaningless." I bury the lunchbox deep in the pantry, devastated to imagine he may never joyfully carry it again.

I realize I'm experiencing the same emotions as the five stages of grief: anger first, with denial quickly following. Every morning after waking, I keep my eyes closed and pray that the entire thing is a bad dream. I hope to find Ross next to me upon opening my eyes, but I am gravely disappointed every time.

And I've already started bargaining too. During Ross's surgery, I return to God. *I'll go to church more often if Ross recovers fully*, I promise. *I'll be a better person.* I've given up alcohol, reasoning if Ross can't celebrate life with a glass of wine, how can I? I've given up formal meals, too, because it doesn't feel right eating without Ross by my side or at a restaurant with other people, no matter how kind their invitations. I eat mainly modest sandwiches at Ross's bedside that I bring from home. It hasn't taken long for me to lose ten pounds.

It also hasn't taken long for me to wonder, after only being married for seven years, if Ross will still recognize me with the trauma his brain has sustained.

FOUR DAYS AFTER surgery, Ross is taken out of sedation and promptly pulls out his endotracheal tube. Amazingly, he can breathe on his own. His voice is weak but it feels like a major triumph to hear it. Tentatively, I lean close to him.

"Ross, do you know who I am?" I ask gently.

He weakly mouths "wife."

That's good, but not enough for me. "Do you know my name?"

"Denise," his gravelly voice ekes out, barely audible.

I let out an exhale of relief.

THE NEXT DAY, Ross pulls out his remaining chest tube himself. The staff rushes to restrain him, but by the time they reach him, he has already accomplished it without causing another collapsed lung, a danger the medical team warned me about if the tube came out prematurely. I understand the nurses' desire to control his actions while he's in the hospital, but my husband has always been a fighter.

At this point, with Ross's limited ability to talk, we attempt communication by other means. The first thing he does is spell a word on his thigh with his index finger: "Hell."

My heart aches when I see this. I can only imagine how trapped he must feel and it's killing me. I know he needs to be able to express himself, so I ask him if he thinks he can write. He nods, so I find some paper. He is so weak that he's barely able to hold a pen, but after a few attempts, I discover that if I move the paper as he writes, I can decipher his scribbles.

"Too drugged. Feel drunk," he scrawls.

More words that alarm me.

But now that he seems to be making some progress, I'm hopeful they'll dial down the narcotics so that he won't feel so drugged from here on out—and that the hell he's experiencing will soon be a distant memory.

THOUGH WE WERE encouraged in the beginning, Ross is having more and more difficulty breathing. His oxygen saturation is slowly declining and he becomes paler and weaker every day. The physicians in the ICU inform me they are not optimistic that he'll be able to breathe on his own much longer. I am barely digesting this when all the alarms begin screaming. Nurses rush in and I am quickly escorted out of the room with Ross's mother. The commotion makes me dizzy as I try to see what's happening. But in a flash, the medical team pulls the curtains shut.

Ross's mother is alarmingly calm, saying things will be fine, but I start to silently, tearfully, strike a deal with God.

◆

chapter seven

ROSS

Sleep Deprivation

I t is impossible to sleep well in the ICU. The beeping and buzzing alone is enough to drive anyone crazy. Noises emanate from nearly all the equipment. Some are alarms; others are status updates. Regardless, these noises chase sleep away.

If I do happen to drift off, it doesn't last. If I'm not awakened by the machines, I'm startled awake every hour by a well-intentioned nurse. Checking tubes, tightening restraints, adjusting settings. There is always a pair of hands poking or prodding. It feels like a cutaneous invasion.

And then there is the intermittent squeezing.

The pneumatic cuff crawls along my upper arm every thirty minutes, completely occluding blood flow to measure my systolic blood pressure. This alternates with what feels like a giant wrestler putting a death grip on my calves. The systemic compression devices affixed to both my legs blow up to high pressure every several minutes throughout the night to decrease the risk of blood clots. Though I know how important this is—clots can travel to the lungs and block oxygenation, killing me in an instant—I silently scream for the squeezing to stop.

This all occurs in a bed that should at the very least be

comfortable. But it's not. It is rigid, firm, noisy. Even if I had a chance of finding a comfortable position, which is impossible with the restraints, lines, tubes, and numerous broken ribs, the pads that soak up seepage of my bodily fluids bunch and gather underneath me.

And the wires. The seemingly endless miles of wires attached to sensors on my body to transmit vital data. They feel like they're everywhere, draped over my limbs, painfully tugging my skin. Even worse, they easily wrap around body parts and can strangulate if no one's present to prevent it.

This anti-sleep environment in the ICU makes no sense. It is the exact opposite of what I need, of what anyone needs, for a healthy recovery. The lack of restorative rest is adding to my confusion and delirium. It is no surprise that the only way I can sleep at all is with strong medications, yet piling on the narcotics only makes it worse.

chapter eight

ROSS

Communication

After I extubated myself, they restrained me—"restrained" being a nice word for "tied down." Then I crashed from my inability to breathe, and they intubated me all over again. Restraints are barbaric. They're tight. They hurt. The endotracheal tube feels like a garden hose down my throat. It blocks my vocal cords as it enters my lungs, so I have no way of verbalizing anything, and enunciation with my lips is impossible. Imagine lying in bed, fully aware, and not being able to speak, to move, to scratch your own itch. Being in this state makes me feel isolated, imprisoned, alone—and, at times, abandoned even.

To get people's attention, I've resorted to the only thing I *can* do: snap my fingers.

"Don't think I'll come running if you snap once you're home," Denise teases.

But the nurses aren't as amused as my wife. In fact, they become skilled at ignoring my snaps, looking in another direction, or making eye contact with me but walking right past without stopping. I realize it might seem annoying to them, but they clearly have no idea how unbearable it is to feel this helpless.

I'm so desperate for loving human contact that I request multiple times that Denise climb into bed with me. Of course, it is not allowed. I am so utterly miserable in my aloneness that Denise instead offers to rub my feet. This simple massage, this gesture of love, transports me. It is so comforting to feel her touch this way that I wish with my whole being that she never had to stop.

I'VE NOW BECOME aware of numbness—or what is called dorsal ulnar cutaneous neuropraxia—in my left arm and hand, but I have no way of telling my doctors this is happening. As a surgeon, I know the nerve has likely been damaged by either the persistent swelling of my arm from the trauma, or the restraints that are too tight, or both. I also know the nerve might regenerate since it was never severed, but I strongly suspect it is the restraints that have caused the specific nerve to be injured, not merely edema. I'm grateful it's my non-dominant arm, but I'm frustrated that no one is addressing it, and that the pins and needles often awaken me during my infrequent sleep.

In one of my brief lucid moments, I want to touch the tube entering my mouth. I know what being intubated means, of course, but I still can't fathom how I've ended up in my current situation. In a truly romantic gesture, Denise releases my hand restraints over the protests of my mother. She lets me trace the tube with my hand up to my mouth. This is when I begin to process the gravity of my situation.

It is a veritable nightmare I've been drifting in and out of for days.

NOW THAT I'M able to write, with Denise feeding the paper under the pen like a printer, I'm grateful for a way to communicate. But it is a monumental task, made worse by being hampered with the restraints. Because I'm so weak, Denise encourages me to write in block, not cursive, thinking it will be easier. Either way, I inevitably run out of steam at the most critical point. I often write "I need . . ." and the rest is illegible. I don't know why I feel the need to write in complete sentences when I don't have the energy to finish them.

Finally, Denise says, "Just write one word, the word that matters most to you, and we'll go from there."

I write the same words over and over again. *Water. Leave. Pee.*

I have a catheter, but it makes me feel like my bladder is full despite it being drained. There is also a deep burning at the base of my penis. This catheter was invented in 1937 and has barely changed in the eighty years since. I've heard hundreds of patients throughout my career say they needed to urinate despite the catheter draining their bladder. I've also heard nurses across the world reply, "You have a bladder catheter, so don't worry about it."

Now I know why these platitudes frustrate patients so much. The nurses have no idea what it feels like.

I add it to my mental list of things I want to champion for change when I get out of here, and drift back into a drug-induced fog.

◆

chapter nine

ROSS

Escape

I have no idea how long I've been here. I only know I feel like I'm in prison. Where else do you get physically tortured and mentally ignored? The line between a hospital and jail is hard to discern. I've tried to cooperate but I know too much from the physician's side. This is why doctors get a bad rap for being difficult patients. But I don't care about that. All I care about is escaping this place. I know my body is broken right now, but in my mind, I feel well, and I desperately want to be in control of my own destiny. I've already pulled tubes from my body I felt I didn't need anymore. Now I want to walk and feel free.

On more than one occasion, when Denise has been at my side, I've pointed to the door and gesticulated frantically, making my index and middle fingers walk toward the door like the old Yellow Pages advertisements.

"You want to leave?" she'd ask, already knowing the answer.

I would nod my head vigorously.

"But we've talked about this," she'd say gently. "How would we successfully manage that with you on the ventilator?"

I'd simply raise both my arms in a shrug and wave off this fact.

"I know you're frustrated, babe." She'd furrow her brow in solidarity with me. "We'll see what tomorrow brings, okay?"

But tomorrow never came fast enough.

IT'S ABOUT A week after my rib plating, and I'm off the ventilator once again. Denise needs a much-deserved break; she wants to help the boys pack for their return to school, and I whisper that I understand. My parents offer to stay with me, so Denise kisses me, promises to be back soon, and leaves. I can tell my parents don't feel much need to babysit me, so after only a short time, they announce that they're hungry and are going out to get some food. They appear wholly unconcerned about leaving me alone as I watch them disappear from the ICU.

I glance around. No nurses or staff are nearby. I am not tied down. Now is my chance.

I somehow sit up among all the lines and wires and swing my legs over the edge of the bed. I drop my feet to the floor and try to stand, but I am so weak that my legs buckle and I fall face-first to the floor. Almost immediately, staff swarms around me, clearly upset. "How could this have happened?" they ask me. "Does anything hurt?" I am now thoroughly confused since, in my mind, all I was doing was leaving this unpleasant place.

In an instant I am whisked off for yet another head CT to make sure there is no damage. Once again, I am lucky. No broken bones or teeth. Maybe someone is watching over me, or all the prayers are indeed being heard.

Perhaps the biggest irony is how fervently I have fought in my career for a reduction in patient falls. When I first arrived, a nearby ICU nurses' break room boasted there had been over "245 days since the last patient fall."

I managed to end that streak.

chapter ten

DENISE

Withdrawal

A lthough they say it's for his safety, it pains me to see Ross tied to the hospital bed. After his attempted escape, they put him back on periodic sedation and into full-time restraints so that he can't pull out any more tubes.

A doctor appears at Ross's bedside. "At this point," he says to me with a grand sigh, "I recommend a tracheostomy and feeding tube."

My favorite trauma surgeon, the one who did two tours in Afghanistan, is off duty. It is his covering surgeon who makes the recommendation, explaining that prolonged placement of the endotracheal tube through the vocal cords can lead to necrosis of important internal throat tissue from the unrelieved pressure. "But just so you're aware, once we do the tracheostomy, Ross will physically lose the ability to use his voice. Air will reach the lungs, but because the tracheostomy sits below the vocal cords, air won't flow into the larynx."

I agree that it makes sense to relieve that pressure, but I'm concerned about Ross going through yet another procedure. I am also worried about the visible scar it will leave and wonder if it's all necessary. The irony of Ross, a former ENT resident, needing a trach is not lost on me, and I hope he'll be breathing on his own soon enough not to have to endure one.

But Ross is apparently lucid enough to chime in and gives a literal thumbs up.

"See?" the doctor says. "Even Ross thinks it's a good idea."

I'm not sure I can trust Ross's judgment at this point; he will say anything to be relieved of the endotracheal tube. But not having a crystal ball to know what's best, I discuss it with my in-laws and John—Ross's trusted friend/mentor from Iowa whom we recently saw at a plastic surgery meeting in Miami one month before Ross's fall—then sign the consent form.

AT THIS POINT, I am justifiably concerned about Ross becoming addicted to opioids. People of all racial and educational backgrounds have become addicted to narcotics after hospitalization in our country, and I am haunted by Ross scrawling out, "too drugged." I know he wants the amount decreased, and so do I, but asking the ICU team to do that, especially after the stunt he pulled trying to escape, is no easy feat. Keeping him sedated is in the best interest of the healthcare team, as it keeps their jobs easier at night if Ross is docile. Sometimes caregivers are more worried about patients complaining of pain than they are about lessening it a little. Of course, no one wants to experience pain, and decreasing pain is important, but it is part of the healing process. Why do we believe the complete absence of pain is the goal? We need to rethink this belief, especially considering the danger of lifelong addiction to drugs used to mitigate pain.

I've become increasingly annoyed arriving each morning and being told that Ross was "agitated" at night and required increased narcotic dosing to calm down. This makes no sense. During the day, he is monitored and calm with me at his side.

Why is he so different at night? I'm convinced that administering narcotics for "agitation," particularly at night, is one of the biggest problems in the ICU. How can a patient not be agitated with the endless sleep interruptions, untold discomforts, and incessant buzzing and beeping of machines?

I begin hounding the ICU team about it, begging that they stop these addictive medications. I also remind them it's been proven that reparative brain healing can't properly occur in drug-induced sleep. Luckily, the wonderful lead trauma doctor understands my concerns and removes the "as needed" order. After that, Ross starts becoming more lucid.

I WON'T PRETEND I'm not thrilled and relieved that Ross is being weaned off the sedatives, but I hadn't considered that he might go through drug withdrawals. I first notice he has tremors. Then he has a low-grade fever.

"Are these withdrawal symptoms?" I ask the nurses.

"Probably," they confirm.

I'm now certain that if I hadn't insisted on stopping the narcotics that kept Ross sedated while on the ventilator, he could have survived a devastating trauma only to be incapacitated by secondary effects of the drugs—drugs used to keep him "comfortable."

I HAVE COME to fear that Ross is merely a broken body to everyone. I understand that keeping him alive is their assignment for that day, which they are accomplishing well. Some take the time to ask how I am doing and offer support. But mentally and emotionally, I am bereft. I feel completely alone. Until Ross is back to full capacity, this is my problem alone to manage.

chapter eleven

ROSS

Hygiene

My mouth feels like a cobblestone road covered by a swamp. Not one nurse has brushed my teeth since I've been in the ICU. I am labeled as "NPO" (nothing to eat), so all I get is an occasional swabbing inside my mouth with a green sponge on a lollipop stick, which nurses wet with a few drops of water. It's ridiculous to think this quenches any level of thirst or moistens my mouth. The fact is, it's only a tease and does nothing to comfort me. Even worse, it tastes like chemicals.

I am appalled that there is no dental hygiene. Even though it would be challenging to clean a patient's teeth with an endotracheal tube in the way, I don't think anyone receives attention to their teeth. Yes, they're keeping me alive, but I can't help but wonder how many cavities and root canals people need as a result of modern medicine ignoring this critical daily routine.

Just days before I got here, I was dealing with an infected, slightly mobile molar. My dentist was pessimistic about his ability to save the tooth, so he had his hygienist deep clean it and hoped for the best. I admit I'm amazed I'm not feeling pain in this tooth. I suspect the antibiotics I received when I had pneumonia may have helped. Also, since I haven't eaten, there's been less bacterial load in my mouth—and I haven't upset the tooth by chewing. Still, the whole idea of my mouth not being clean for weeks is a travesty.

BODILY WASTE IS an entirely other matter.

I am relieved when they finally remove the bladder catheter, but this means I must now carefully urinate into a plastic jug— the twenty-first-century answer for managing urine if you can't get out of bed.

Problem one is the jug design. My penis is so shriveled from disuse that peeing into the jug is an acrobatic challenge. After dribbling everywhere, what ends up in the urinal is then easily spilled on me as I struggle to place the jug on the side of the bed.

Problem two is germs. I'm always wondering whether the plastic urinal was previously used by someone and not cleaned afterward. Resting my penis along the plastic lip of the urinal, I can only hope it is unused.

Problem three is positioning. I have to accomplish all of this while lying completely flat on my back.

Defecating is another pleasure.

Though I haven't had solid food in weeks, it's still necessary to move my bowels from time to time. The bedpan is a poorly designed device, dating back millennia. When I can manage to maneuver it under myself to "sit" on it, my butt cheeks hurt significantly. I might move my bowels, but all I can think is, *How am going to wipe myself?* It is nearly impossible due to immobility, pain, or just simple physics.

I always hope the next time I have to go I'll be stronger. I cringe having my buttocks wiped by a stranger. But every time I attempt to do it myself, my arms are so weak that I can't lift myself to do it.

I don't know who's more humiliated, the poor technician or me.

◆

chapter twelve

DENISE

Transfer

F ive days after receiving the tracheostomy and gastrostomy tube, Ross is transferred out of the ICU and into a step-down unit—a location in the hospital where they provide an intermediate level of care between the ICU and the general medical-surgical wards. He is thankfully off the ventilator but on something known as a biPAP—bilevel positive airway pressure—that helps keep his lungs aerated. He doesn't need a tracheostomy for this, as there are machines that can perform this through the mouth, but they use the tracheal opening nonetheless. The tracheostomy also serves as a safety net if Ross fatigues again from breathing. When this doesn't occur, I start to question the necessity of the tracheostomy and, worse, blame myself for some of his suffering since I provided consent for this procedure.

It is here in the step-down unit that Ross is now able to talk with a device called a cap. Previously, he could only form words with his dry lips without any sound at all. The fact that we've been able to communicate that way is a testament to our simpatico relationship. But now, with the cap sitting over the tracheostomy, Ross can actually say words. His voice is hoarse and weak, but hearing him say "I love you" in his breathy staccato voice is an unimaginable gift.

"I'm starting to become a human being again," he says, and tears immediately well in my eyes.

Ross also expresses his intense desire for liquid.

"I crave seltzer," he says. "I need seltzer."

He tells me how he fantasizes about the bottle, the fizz, and the quenching of his thirst. He starts negotiating with the trauma service during their rounds, targeting the youngest and most sympathetic-looking member of the trauma team. He is so desperate that he offers a scholarship in the name of whomever brings him a seltzer. He then begs members of the ICU team, who convey it to the trauma team, who defer to the GI team. They eventually conference and agree after Ross pushes hard. Being a physician in this instance helps move the process along.

The following morning, the youngest member of the trauma team brings a seltzer from a local bodega. Ross is so overjoyed that I wouldn't have been surprised if he kissed the young man.

A nurse doles out a few drops in a cap. "Small sips only," she says. "No more than a few ounces a day."

Though she watches him like a hawk as he indulges, it is as if the bubbles are bringing Ross back to life.

It is also here that Ross finally receives his first shave in weeks. He looks so old in the hospital bed, with his gray beard and hanging skin due to wasting muscles. The nurse sincerely sympathizes with Ross's pain and wishes to transform him back to his former self. but instead of it being a pleasant experience with some soft, nice-smelling foam, the nurse tries her best to carefully shave him dry. I can see Ross's discomfort as she edges the newly grown beard off his chin, and as I notice the redness of his skin, I begin to stop her. But Ross tells me with his eyes to stay as silent as he is, to just be grateful he's alive.

The step-down unit is where I also realize that we are not the only ones making this difficult journey. As a hospital providing charity care to all people in need within this large city, a diversity of cultures is represented. Ross now has roommates, many of whom he would never have seen otherwise. I see family members visiting their loved ones, some clothed in hijabs and others in yarmulkes. What we all have in common is that we are suffering the same immense pain and fear for our loved ones.

Unfortunately, Ross is experiencing illusions as a side effect of the narcotics. "I see floating strings everywhere," he tells me. "Everyone has gossamer coming from their right shoulders that trails off into the distance." He further tells me that some people have random strings poking out beyond their hair, and that it's very difficult for him to know what's real.

"Don't tell anyone else," I whisper. Maybe I'm being paranoid, but I'm determined not to let anything land him back in the ICU, which would be a step backward. I'm now firm about getting Ross to the next level of care and in a rehab facility, painfully aware that the longer he languishes in a hospital, the greater the risk of his suffering a hospital-acquired infection or another patient fall.

AFTER PUSHING HARD for four days—making daily calls to our insurance company and coordinating efforts between the hospital case worker and the rehab facility's admissions manager—Ross is finally approved for transfer to a rehabilitation facility. I continue to argue that his chances of a complication remain high if he stays in an acute-care facility, and I know that rehab is the next important step in getting our lives back to normal.

But just as we are about to initiate the transfer, we get deflating news: his hematocrit (blood level) test came back a little low.

"Can you just repeat the test?" I ask. "You know how it can fluctuate."

The next day, Ross's hematocrit hits the acceptable minimal level. I insist on his transfer and after some hours of pushback, they finally pack him into an ambulance for transport.

ARRIVING AT THE rehabilitation facility should be a joyous milestone—yet it's anything but. Everywhere I turn, Ross's fellow patients are the story of what could have been. People with severe brain injuries and paralysis are his new roommates, and everyone is issued a wheelchair with a headrest, regardless of their strength and mobility. Certainly Ross needs a lot of strengthening, but to see him in the same chair as a quadriplegic is frightening. Sadly, some of the patients in this facility have experienced brain swelling from their injuries, the same diagnosis Ross miraculously escaped. Because of this, they wear helmets to protect their brains, which are sitting just below the scalp without bone. Being surrounded by these individuals could bring Ross down, but to his credit, he remains chipper and more determined than ever to beat the odds.

Fighter that he is, Ross pushes hard through his therapies. But on his fourth day, after the patient-care tech carefully places him on the commode and pulls a curtain, Ross asks for more privacy since I am nearby. Instead of leaving, though, I clandestinely sit at the end of the curtain, pretending I am reading a newspaper. Thankfully, I notice from the corner of my eye when Ross starts to drift backward and quickly leap to catch him before he falls hard to the floor. The tech arrives within seconds after I call for help, but the truth is, I have stopped another preventable fall.

An evaluation finds that Ross's hematocrit has now dropped to dangerously low levels, so the rehab facility has no choice but to transfer him back to the trauma center. We have now taken the step backward that I feared.

After receiving multiple blood transfusions, the physicians at the trauma hospital suspect bleeding from a stress ulcer and confirm the diagnosis through an endoscopy. Though the hospital had taken measures to prevent this, Ross still developed bleeding ulcers as a result of the stresses in the ICU. His gastrointestinal physician places hemostatic clips in his stomach and small bowel, which are used to prevent bleeding in the GI tract, and tells me Ross will need to take acid blockers for three months—a protocol that comes with a host of potentially detrimental side effects, but the doctors believe the benefits outweigh the risks.

After spending four more days in the same step-down unit as before at the trauma center—and after endless urging from Ross—they finally remove his tracheostomy since he no longer needs any support for breathing, and he is once again transferred to the rehabilitation facility for what we hope will be his last stop before coming home with me for good.

ROAD TO
RECOVERY

◆

chapter thirteen

ROSS

Rehab

I am determined to conquer rehab as quickly as possible and get back to my life. In my mind's eye, I'm still the man I was when I fell that day in December, only with a few substantial challenges to overcome.

For starters, staying immobilized in an ICU bed for three weeks caused severe negative nitrogen balance. Despite IV lines and feeding tubes, not getting exercise meant my body cannibalized itself, breaking down my muscles for energy. What muscles remained were severely weakened from lack of use, including the accessory breathing muscles of my neck from being on the ventilator. Once I was off it, I was out of breath and shaky just shuffling twenty feet with a walker. I felt like an astronaut returning to Earth's gravity after months in space—but at least they get to exercise. Trying to project positivity through the pain, I gave a thumb's up and yelled "freedom!" through my capped tracheostomy as I tottered past the nurses' desk.

The physicians saved my life for which I am very grateful, but now that I'm here in rehab, there's no doubt I have an enormous amount of work to do to restore my muscle strength. I can hardly hold my head up or even turn it. Brushing my teeth is painful and exhausting—my arms feel like they weigh hundreds of pounds, and I can barely keep the toothbrush against my teeth, let alone raise my arm to comb my hair. *How will I tie my surgical mask and hat when I return to work?* I wonder. Chewing is extremely difficult, and swallowing after having the trach is even worse. And sneezing? With all the plates in my sternum, a single sneeze causes pain more severe than anything to date.

Despite all this, I keep telling myself it is only a matter of time before I'm the strong, vibrant man I was only one month ago. I know I'm weaker than I ever imagined possible, but it's not until I catch my reflection in a mirror do I realize how far I truly have to go.

Shortly after arriving, I'm elated to learn I'll be receiving my first shower in over a month. After the incessant poking, prodding, and testing I've endured in the ICU, I am no longer shy undressing in front of the technician. My biggest concern, after thinning out in the ICU, is freezing to death. But that is eclipsed when I see myself for the first time since the accident.

"What the fuck?!" I blurt out to the mirror, completely taken aback.

My paternal grandfather seems to be staring back at me. I have his loose neck skin, gaunt cachectic look, and sunken eyes. I knew I'd lost *some* weight, but it looks as though I've lost at least thirty pounds the way my skin hangs off my bones. An IV dangles down my side, and unsightly caps cover my tracheostomy and gastrostomy. But perhaps most alarming is the long, red snake of a scar slicing from my nipple and wrapping around my flank, then traveling to my spine. It makes me look like I was split in half and put together again.

"You okay?" the technician, Maurice, asks.

I muster half a head shake. Words escape me. I'm certain

Maurice has seen it all, but I can't fathom how the "me" I've envisioned has morphed nearly beyond recognition.

"The shower should be nice, Dr. Z.," he says, trying to placate me.

I've asked everyone to call me Ross, as I do not like the hierarchy a title creates, but Maurice prefers to use a modicum of formality.

I nod weakly, steadying myself after the shock I've received, as Maurice eases me into the shower chair. He tests the water to make sure it will be a comfortable temperature before gently directing it toward me. When he does, the water feels magical pouring over my body. I realize in that moment it is the first familiar thing I'm experiencing since my fall, and I desperately want to stand and enjoy the simple gift of soaping and rinsing myself. But I am too weak to stand and must be satisfied with my accompanied sit-down shower. I close my eyes and revel in what feels like a milestone in my journey back to normalcy as Maurice gingerly lathers one body part at a time.

When I'm washed as well as I can be, Maurice carefully pats me dry, being mindful of all my tender incisions. I still feel damp in spots, but I can't remember feeling more refreshed in a very long time.

AS I BEGIN my physical therapy in earnest, everyone—except Denise—states emphatically to me that I won't be able to return to work until late spring or early summer, and that's at the soonest.

I can't blame them for seeing a long road ahead for me. How can they not when I have so many limitations. Even gaining weight seems impossible when I can barely swallow food that has no taste to me and when I feel full after only two bites. Still, this prediction simply feels wrong.

"It won't be that long for me," I tell each of them with conviction. "I'll be back to work by late February."

Over and over again, I see eyebrows raised, hear words to the contrary.

But they don't know me.

I visualize returning to work within a month. I picture my office in my head and see myself there doing my daily duties. I imagine performing surgeries and seeing patients for pre- and post-op appointments. Every day, every minute, I do something to achieve my goal. Even while sitting in bed, I do some type of physical exercise. I have to. Right now, rehab activities like climbing stairs or carrying a glass filled with water for 100 feet are Herculean tasks; it requires intense focus to push through these simple acts centered on basic skills, gross balance, and strength. It commands equal fortitude to walk the hallways and turn my head to the left and right, not to mention simulating placing groceries on shelves. Each undertaking leaves me shaky and weak; every muscle aches from the slightest bit of movement. Even standing up straight is difficult and I worry I'll develop a permanent hunchback. I'm so exhausted from these mild exercises that I need to nap during the afternoon.

Still, I never lose sight of—or belief in—my goal.

Specially trained therapists also work on my cognitive skills. In a room surrounded by stroke victims who cannot speak—or who can communicate only by painstakingly tapping out a text message—I'm asked to solve puzzles. I feel like I'm living in *One Flew Over the Cuckoo's Nest*, it is such a strange and depressing environment. I am quizzed daily on facts. I'm asked to remember sequences of numbers and items. One cognitive therapist, Fred, graciously allows me to talk about my love of Roman history. The next day, we practice booking vacations on airlines and plan theoretical trips online.

Fred tests me frequently to attempt to "score" my recovery. As a physician, I know the significance of the mental status tests everyone persistently administers: draw a clock, recall words, name certain animals. The fact that I went to Harvard and Yale is now completely meaningless. I'm merely a patient labeled with a brain injury.

One might think I look forward to weekends, when the facility schedules no therapies and I have a reprieve from the arduous effort I put forth hours each day. Instead, I'm baffled by this and wonder why they don't hire more people to fill the empty shifts. I don't see the lull as a break, but rather a hindrance to my recovery. So, I facilitate my own therapy protocols; I try to use my arms to propel my wheelchair instead of being pushed. Rather than passively watching Netflix or Hulu, I perform mental tasks and play memory games. In doing so, I can literally feel my brain synapses working to recover. When I first arrived at rehab, I couldn't remember my home address, but a blurry 820 has become a crisp 876 within a matter of days. Blessed with not having a severed spinal cord or a damaged brain, there is no way I will waste the miraculous gift I've been given by becoming passive in my recovery.

I got a second chance at life.

Predictions be damned.

I will beat this.

ALTHOUGH EATING IS a chore with little enjoyment because of my malfunctioning taste buds and difficulty swallowing, I'm craving what I call "old man Jewish food"—perhaps because I'm turning into one. When my brother visits me and asks what foods I'd like, I order liver and tongue. To the untrained, these are disgusting foods, but for some reason, I find them delicious, probably because they are more about texture than taste. Texture is all I can discern at this point, either from prolonged intubation, desiccation of my tongue, my temporal bone fracture, or some combination of the three. Brett not only indulges my odd request but makes liver and tongue sandwiches for me at my bedside since I'm too weak to do it myself.

"I can't even open a bottle of Ensure without help," I joke.

Brett and Denise just shake their heads.

"I had a call with a time-share agent earlier today and he offered me the deal of a lifetime." I wait a beat. "I couldn't resist investing in it."

Denise is not amused.

ONE OF THE nicest differences between the hospital and the rehab facility is being able to positively interact with the staff. In the ICU, I was either too drugged or too hindered to do anything much but feel like a science experiment. But here, I get to engage my brain and talk to a slew of remarkable employees, many of whom are eager to share what it's really like to be in their jobs.

Vanessa, one of the most vivacious people I've ever met, tells me about the racism she encounters. "It's sad," she says. "An older patient may not trust me because I'm black, or they might call me a derogatory name."

I shake my head, incredulous. I can't believe it's the year 2019 and we're having this conversation. "I'm so sorry," I say. "You don't deserve that."

She shrugs. "I agree. But some people are still stuck in a different way of thinking."

Then there's Renee, who takes so much pride in her outstanding work.

"How many people did you bathe today?" I ask, making casual conversation.

"Oh," she says, "I'm not allowed to discuss that."

I furrow my brow. "Really?"

She nods. I find it interesting, and frankly ridiculous, how the corporate spin permeates every level of care to the point that a tech can't even answer an innocent question, one I can't fathom could be twisted to harm anyone in any way.

Maurice, my faithful "shower buddy," cheerfully deals with more than just orchestrating my bathing routine.

"What's that in your ear?" he asks me on one of my first days here.

I lightly shrug. "I have no idea."

The next thing I know, he's extracted an old blood clot the size of an engorged leech. I cringe but he simply laughs it off and tells me this is part of recovery.

Another day I tell him I'm worried I might have a bowel accident as I settle onto the shower seat.

"No worries," he says cheerfully. "If you do, at least we're here in the shower."

"That's true," I say with a laugh that echoes his.

When Maurice isn't working, there's Georgette, quiet but strong and keeps her word. We set a time for a shower and she is there.

And I could never forget Morris, who gave me my first scalp haircut. As he clipped and shaved, I remember being moved when he said, "I owe my career success to my wife and mom."

As my foggy hospital memories become clearer, one more person materializes in my mind:

Maria, who worked in environmental services at the trauma hospital, would notice Denise at my bedside every morning. Not wanting to disturb us, she started arriving fifteen minutes earlier each day to clean my bay. "How's your husband?" she would ask whenever she saw Denise. "He looks better every day!" By the time I could talk around the tracheostomy, Maria had convinced me to take her salsa dancing after my discharge.

Each of these self-sacrificing people, with their kind hearts and sincere compassion, makes an indelible mark on me and undeniably helps to renew my waning faith in the medical profession.

AS MUCH AS I relish being out of the ICU and the step-down unit, and having a much more relaxed atmosphere during the day, evenings in the rehab facility can be scary. I'm so out of the habit of getting restful sleep that I lie awake staring at the clock, my roommate's labored breathing an annoying soundtrack in the darkness, as I'm plagued with a barrage of questions from my monkey mind in contrast to my optimistic one.

I've faced death and escaped, but will I really fully recover?

How will I go back to work?

Will I ever truly regain my strength?

When will I have the dexterity to operate again?

Will my patients trust that I'm fine to take care of them?

And I thought I'd be untethered here at night, but some of the night technicians are so focused on simply getting through their shift without any issues that they put us in literal lockdown. On those nights, the technician lifts the side rails of the bed and traps us like caged animals. If anyone is still too active, they are physically restrained and given drugs to knock them out for the night. I find it reprehensible to be treated this way. But if there's a fall, we hear "Dr. Tripp" called on the paging system—code for "someone's down." The legal and professional fallout can be so significant when this happens that there are those who simply don't want to risk anything.

With so many patients having poor ambulation skills, the facility has a means of labeling the level of risk: the color of the socks we're given reflects our freedom ranking. My yellow ones signify that I require supervision when walking. In other words, I've been reduced to a "less-than-able-bodied" individual, a label I resent. They have no idea what this does to a patient mentally. If a person takes this in, they may believe they'll never get past that stage. I understand I'm too weak right now to walk unattended, but I also can't help but wonder if this label is for my own protection or if a corporate lawyer is protecting "the system."

In all fairness to the facility, though, patients do try to escape. Some are confused and wander off accidentally, while others feel like prisoners and dream of home. I strongly relate to the latter category, but the facility cannot just "lose" a patient, so the employees prep for breakouts like prison guards. If someone gets out, another coded page comes over the intercom: "Dr. Departo." It's not funny, I know, but when I feel like being a troublemaker, I tell a nurse or unit secretary that I'm looking for Dr. Departo. It rarely elicits the response I hope for, but I get a kick out of it every time.

One night, I summon one of the techs, Antonio.

"Hey," I whisper. "If you don't raise my bedrails, I promise not to get up unattended."

He's aware of my track record as a bit of a jokester and seems hesitant to cut a deal with me. But when I tell him I know he's taking a big chance on me, he trusts my promise—and I keep it.

When he checks on me hours later, his smile signifies our mutual respect and makes me feel I've witnessed humanity at its best in this web of corporate-governed medical madness.

A FEW NIGHTS later, I'm still awake at 3:00 a.m. Denise has wrangled me a single room, but even though it's quieter, I'm restless with my mind abuzz. Vanessa is on duty, and when she comes by for her rounds, I beg her to take me for a walk. Even though I'm not cleared to walk far distances, Vanessa feels sympathy for me. So we quietly saddle up the wheelchair and tour the facility like kids who've sneaked out of the house without our parents knowing. When we reach the sunroom, a nurse named Michael is there.

He gives us a tsk-tsk look. "What are you two up to?" he says with a chuckle.

"This one can't sleep," Vanessa says. "So we're just taking a little stroll."

"Ahh . . . well, roll on over."

Vanessa parks me next to Michael and we immediately fall into an intense discussion about the pharmaco-industrial complex. Just a doctor and a nurse, freely expressing our concerns about the profession we love and where we fear it's going. It is wonderful to be able to speak openly to each other, but more than that, it is another pocket of time in which I feel a surge of gratitude. The human-to-human interaction is desperately needed in medicine, and there is not enough of it. Michael could have insisted Vanessa take me back to my room, but he didn't. Vanessa could have tethered me to my bed knowing I wasn't sleeping, but she didn't. Instead, she took the time to listen to me and relieve some of my anxiety. She and Michael didn't know it, but that night, they made my life feel worth living.

ON FEBRUARY 1, 2019, fewer than two weeks into my recu-
peration at in-patient rehab, something that's been brewing
finally comes to a head: tension that can no longer be ignored
causes an irreparable schism with my parents.

Many physicians are used to pontificating rather than
questioning, to giving their opinion rather than actively listening. It's easy for them to mentally avoid difficult situations by
hiding behind so-called facts. Sadly, this is precisely what I face
whenever my parents come for a visit.

Despite my debilitated physical appearance, there is objective evidence of my improvement: I can move all four limbs. I
can feel my brain seeking out the proper neural pathways, and
facts previously lost to me are crystalizing rapidly. Yet I am
gravely hurt and disappointed that my parents don't see me for
what I can do. Instead of expressing hope and encouragement
for overcoming my condition, they express a form of resignation, blindly repeating their conditioned response and continuing to define me as an injured, cachectic patient who has a
long road to recovery. It feels like suffocation, this refusal to
echo my optimism and my goal of returning home and to work
sooner than anyone imagines, and it overshadows my recovery.

Over and over, I've observed that the technicians caring
for me in rehab, most of whom hail from either the Caribbean
islands or the inner city, express more faith in me—and their
deep faith in God's desire to help me heal—than my own parents do. And these techs are strangers. They have no connection to me personally. Yet they are my cheerleaders. If they
doubt I can meet my goal, they no longer say so.

At one point, my father asked to see my initial radiologic
images from the day I fell, presumably to see the details of my
temporal bone fracture. But that had been several weeks ago.
When Denise and I ask him to return the disks—which, after

all, are part of my personal health information—he is hurt. I don't know if he's interpreted the request as my not trusting him, but regardless of my reasons, he is not in a position to refuse. When he reluctantly surrenders the disks as I started to recover, having my mother perfunctorily deliver them to me, he makes it extraordinarily clear that our relationship will be irrevocably changed.

I've come to realize that I may have no choice in who surrounds me in rehab, but I do have a choice in whom I invite in from the outside to participate in my healing journey. I repeatedly invite my parents to actively join me, but they refuse. This unnecessary fissure that has formed in my family is tragic and sad, but at the present moment, I have greater things to put my focus toward.

WHEN FEBRUARY 3RD arrives, the facility is buzzing with excitement. It's Super Bowl Sunday, and families and patients gather around the television in the sunroom as if it's the biggest event in history. Two young-adult patients with head injuries from car accidents, with their shaved heads and corked tracheostomies, sit across from me in their wheelchairs. An older patient who suffered a stroke is planted near me in his wheelchair. The visiting families bring wings, soda, and other nutritionally devoid foods for their loved ones, attempting to create some semblance of "fun." And while a feeling of celebration fills the room, so does a sense of gloom. Every single patient in the room appears to have a long road ahead—everyone except for me.

When I arrived, I was too weak to walk long distances and was forced to be wheeled everywhere. One warm winter day, Denise and I went Dr. Departo on the staff and ventured outside. As we circled the perimeter of the building in my wheelchair, I felt overwhelmingly grateful to be alive and for her to be so lovingly at my side.

"Wouldn't it be ironic," I joke, "if you lost control of my chair, and I died rolling down the hill?"

"Don't even kid about that," Denise had said, feigning seriousness. Then we both burst out laughing.

Soon after, I could get up with some effort from the chair, a feat mixed with both joy and guilt, as I knew many of my brethren in the facility would never be able to stand again.

I had put monumental effort into every therapy and every moment of downtime, eagerly anticipating the day a millennial therapist would finally issue a card allowing me, a fifty-two-year-old man, to walk on my own. And now, little more than two weeks after my arrival—against everyone's expectations but mine and Denise's—I held that card in my hand.

I glance at Denise. "I'm so lucky," I whisper.

And she knows exactly how sincerely I mean it.

◆

chapter fourteen

ROSS

Homeward Bound

I t is February 5th, 2019, my older stepson Sotiri's birthday. After only twelve days in the rehabilitation facility, following my second ICU admission after the GI bleed, I am poised to walk out on my own two feet.

The facility is once again abuzz with excitement, only this time, it's for me. My parents aren't there but my brother has come to wish me well; no one in my presence can believe I've fulfilled my goal of leaving this quickly. I would like to think I've been a role model of positive thinking as I receive countless hugs and words of encouragement from the staff. Two weeks ago, I wouldn't have been able to lift my arms to return those hugs. But now, as I say goodbye to them, I'm flooded with gratitude that I can not only embrace these dear people who've helped me in my healing journey, but offer a last wave to them as I walk toward the exit.

A cool, but not cold, evening greets me as Denise pushes the door open, ending my six-week journey of multiple admissions to the ICU, my two stints in the step-down unit, and nearly two weeks of in-patient rehab. I stop for a moment, tilting my head gently upward to breathe in the air. Denise's car is waiting, and I climb into it, something I couldn't have done on my own even one week prior. As she pulls away from the curb and heads toward the main road, I notice every detail of my surroundings. The streetlights seem so crisp, the car seat feels luxurious, the scenery is beautiful. We stop at a local food store to pick up dinner. When I walk into the market, I stare at the rows of products, feeling like an immigrant newly arrived in America, unable to process the bounty. I tell the teenager working behind the counter what I want, and then add, "I'm happy to be alive. I was in an accident and nearly died, but I'm here."

The kid doesn't skip a beat. "Wow, you look pretty good having survived all that."

I smile. Maybe I no longer look as much like my grandfather as I did two and a half weeks ago.

We continue the trip home, and I marvel at the world like a newborn. When we turn down our street, my heart speeds up. We inch down the block and I feel elation when I see it: our house looks like a surreal, unbelievable dream. All I've wanted for the past six weeks is to come home. Even when we enter the garage and I see the supplies for my roof repair exactly where I left them, the past melts into a horrible but distant memory.

I open the door and ease out of the car. Denise gathers my things as I make my way inside. It is nothing short of magical. Once again, I notice every detail, how vibrant and well placed and sentimental everything seems. I want nothing more than to get into our bed—our soft, comfy bed without monitors or wires. Denise follows behind as I slowly climb the stairs to our room, watching my every step like a hawk so she can swoop in if I lose my balance or collapse from weakness. I sit on the bed, then swivel gingerly and lie down. The feeling is beyond words. This is what Denise and I have spent hours praying for: to be together at home, alive and intact.

The therapists had predicted a prolonged stay based on how I appeared when I arrived, but I proved to them that was an unfair assumption. I may have had trouble doing just about everything at first because of all the muscle wasting, but they didn't know what I was made of. They didn't realize they were labeling me by what others have done in the past with a similar condition, not what I believed I could do. I pushed myself to walk the extra steps, to raise my arms higher, to perform the exercises longer, to execute the toughest tasks with autonomy. I never stopped quizzing myself, testing my memory, engaging in conversation. I befriended many of the nurses and therapists and learned their names, greeting them daily in the hallways. If I'd allowed myself to passively fall into the role of a patient with a specific label, I could have easily taken the months, not weeks, they expected for me to recover. But the physician side of my brain refused to be defined in that manner. As the iconoclast, I willed myself to fight their predictions, to refuse to be defined by the treating physicians and fall into a self-fulfilled negative prophecy. I couldn't help but think how much easier it might have been if they had fed me words from the start that showed they believed in me the same way—how much more encouraging it would be for any patient facing an upward climb back to health.

It's true that my early departure date materialized by both the grace of God and hard work, yet Denise and I still had to fight for my release, convincing the doctors I'd be able to function safely at home. Had we not pushed, I would have remained in rehab until insurance restrictions forced me out many weeks, or even months, later. Sadly, this is the current state of healthcare. Because most facilities are paid based on patient count, and physicians are paid for each patient visit, I can't help but wonder if both are motivated to keep people in the role of patient. Although the physicians truly want their patients to recover, our current system of reimbursement no doubt plays a subconscious role in their decisions. Some people seem to be kicked out of medical facilities too soon to make room for the next person, while others are kept longer than necessary. It's not always clear if it's in the best interest of the patient or the facility why someone comes and goes when they do. In my case, all I know is that the fight to leave was worth it.

AFTER A WONDERFUL night's sleep with Denise by my side, I come downstairs to find hard-boiled eggs peeled and ready for me. These are courtesy of my mother-in-law, who has come to stay with us for a week—and whose sole job is to try to fatten me. She is a fabulous Greek cook, but my taste buds are still misfiring, so I have to miss out on some amazing Mediterranean treats. The hard-boiled eggs are a concession; they are healthy for me and easy to eat. But Denise's mom can't wait for me to enjoy her cooking again. Frankly, neither can I.

For the time being—though I'm mastering how to chew and swallow with my new physiology—I still have to deal with having the abdominal feeding tube. "Just in case," the physicians declared. But I'm convinced that the tube is impeding, not helping, me. Instinctively, I sense that it's pulling my stomach against my abdominal wall, mimicking fullness. Though my stomach is virtually empty, signals are sent from my stomach to my brain, telling it to feel sated, thereby decreasing my overall appetite.

"It's no wonder I can't eat more food," I tell Denise.

She gives credence to my theory, but until I can see the GI physician and insist he remove it, the tube requires a nightly saline flush—a job Denise selflessly assumes, and that makes me feel inadequate. Although I'm strong enough to be home, I'm still too weak to do certain things for myself, and cleaning my feeding tube is one of them. This is when I must remind myself that it could have been so much worse. Denise could have to help me get out of bed and into a wheelchair each morning; she could have to bathe and feed me for the rest of my life. But that's not what happened, and I console myself that this is only temporary as I feel the odd, cool sensation deep in my stomach of the saline flushing through the tube.

PHYSICALLY, IT'S CLEAR I've come a long way, and the rehab therapists certainly helped me get there. But what they didn't teach was perhaps what I—what anyone in those circumstances—needed the most: a philosophical framework to help me manage my new life.

Lucky for me, I had become interested in Stoic philosophy around the time of my trauma, perhaps divinely. The Stoics have only a few central teachings: how unpredictable the world can be; how brief our moment of life is; and how to be steadfast, strong, and in control of oneself. They also advance that the source of our dissatisfaction rests in our impulsive dependency on our reflexive senses rather than logic. Instead of concerning itself with complicated theories about the world, Stoicism strives to help us overcome destructive emotions and act on what can be acted upon. In short, it's built for action, not endless debate.

With these teachings in mind, I focus on the fact that I cannot change the events that landed me where I am, but I *can* control my reaction. I acknowledge that fear and anger are normal, but I also realize I need to discover the grace of my new situation, to be grateful and enjoy life.

Perhaps the greatest epiphany that comes from these beliefs is that I need a way to help my patients understand these things too.

My mindset is: I suffered an accident—an unexpected and

unintentional event resulting in injury. I accept this completely. If I hold on to the anger, it will serve no constructive purpose. I must see the beauty of every day, as it is a gift. Furthermore, I am incredibly fortunate that I'm not irrevocably harmed. This sounds trite but it's true. On some levels, I am the same person I was on December 22, 2018; on others, I'm markedly different. As I consider how profoundly my life has changed in certain ways, I can see the enormous benefits of training physicians in helping their patients see this dichotomy more clearly.

I imagine the mantras that could replace the old, conditioned ones and feel a swell of hope.

Being frustrated serves no constructive purpose.

Be grateful for all you do have.

It is not the world itself that we control but rather our reaction to it.

IT IS ONLY now at home that I fully realize my family spent both Christmas and New Year's at my bedside in a hospital. When I climbed up onto the roof that fateful day, a brightly lit tree surrounded by gifts was the cornerstone of our living room. Now it was as if it had never been there.

"Where are all the gifts?" I ask Denise.

She takes a hesitant breath. "Upstairs, in the attic. There was no way we could open gifts when we didn't know what might happen to you."

I get it. I know I would have done the same thing if the situation were reversed.

"Well," I venture, "I'm home and in one piece. How about opening them now?"

Denise smiles. "You sure you're up to it?"

"Are you kidding?" I say. "I can't think of a better way to celebrate being home and being alive."

My wife flashes an animated grin. "You sit, and I'll be back." With that she drapes a blanket over me and disappears.

I'm so skinny that it hurts to sit; I have no cushioning in my buttocks anymore. And due to my lack of fat insulation, I'm constantly cold. But sitting there under the blanket that Denise laid over me so lovingly, watching her face light up each time she makes a trip up and back, delivering gifts like Santa Claus, makes me forget I feel any discomfort.

"That's all of them," she finally says.

We both sweep our eyes over the pile.

"Open that one," I say, pointing to a medium-size box.

She pulls it to her and unwraps it. The moment she lifts the lid, tears spring to her eyes. Nestled in the box are tumblers with HIS and HERS engraved on them.

She is speechless as she gently wraps her arms around me.

I'm grateful to have the strength to hold her in return.

It is also not lost on me how tragic it would have been for Denise to open that gift had I never made it home.

chapter fifteen

◆

DENISE

Adjustment

All I've wanted for the past many weeks is to have my husband home. I am profoundly happy and grateful that he has not only made it, but that he has recovered far beyond and much faster than what anyone predicted. I'm also painfully aware that we still have a long journey ahead, both physical and mental.

Now that my family leave has expired, I've returned to work, which means I'm filled with an entirely new level of worry about Ross while I'm gone. I brought my wonderful mother to our home under the guise of being Ross's chef while he recuperates, but the truth is, I need her here in case he requires help during the day. I realize how counterproductive it is to focus on fear-based scenarios, but I can't help but be concerned that Ross might fall down the stairs or slip in the shower if I'm not in the house to monitor his every move.

I also desperately need my mother's emotional support, since Ross's parents have refused to visit us after his father stormed out of the rehab room a few days ago. Despite Ross's unflagging belief in his own recovery and his return to work sooner than later, I admit I feel overwhelmed and strongly desire family around me.

Because Ross wants to return to the office as soon as possible and ensure he has a thriving practice to go back to, he needs to review his patients' charts. To facilitate this, I take on coordinating communication between Ross and his office staff, Margaret and Rosie, so that the correct files are pulled and delivered to our home. Ross also needs to start organizing his office finances. As his power of attorney, I've had next to no time to focus on that. Meanwhile, there are multiple follow-up appointments we need to make; transportation to outpatient rehab three days a week to coordinate. Fortunately, Vasili's friend, who's taking a gap year from college, is available to chauffeur Ross to all these appointments while I'm working, since the boys are now back at college.

My recurring thought becomes: *Will our lives ever be normal again?*

AS MUCH AS I try to stay positive, this newness we are facing terrifies me. Similar to after a death, people tend to be there for you right after the loss; when Ross initially returned home, we were swamped with calls of well wishes and drowning in the plethora of food baskets. But this quickly stopped as people slowly and naturally returned to their own lives. Though many of our friends expressed a desire to visit Ross while he lay incapacitated in the ICU, few expressed interest once he was safely home. Our wonderfully thoughtful friend, Ed, has been a welcome exception: he spent the better part of an afternoon with us just days after Ross's return, and it was one of the most gracious acts we've experienced.

Though I'm not proud to admit it, perhaps I feel jaded, whether merited or not, about who has stepped up in our greatest time of need. A profound feeling of loneliness, and feeling the weight of so much change, can do that. I certainly can't blame anyone for returning to their lives, but I also can't help but wish we didn't feel so forgotten at times. While most everyone in our circle has resumed their everyday routines, Ross and I have a whole new set.

As I think about everything that's transpired over the past two months, I find myself trying harder and harder to understand human nature: *Maybe people expressed more willingness to visit Ross in the ICU because seeing the fallen makes them feel better about their own lives. Perhaps, too, there is a morbid curiosity. Either way, I actively forbade visits to the ICU from his friends and colleagues because I didn't want the image of him on a ventilator to be in their mind's eye if Ross didn't make it—and I knew Ross would never have wanted that either. But once we were home, the offers of support diminished—ironically—at the time we actually needed it most. Yet I have to wonder: what more could I have asked for? Is it even fair of me to expect more than what any one person is willing or able to give?*

All I know is, irrational or not, fair or not, these are the feelings I'm grappling with. This is not to say that I'm not supremely grateful for the relatives who've been able to give us so much of their time. My mother and siblings have been extraordinary with their support. Ross's brother, Brett, and his wife, Lori, have also been remarkable. I know we could have never gotten through such a tragic and draining event without the familial love and support we have received from them to give us the strength to continue. But now that Ross is home, it does feel like we are standing at the bottom of a whole new mountain and that we have no one to climb it with but each other.

◆

chapter sixteen

ROSS

Outpatient

N ow that I've officially graduated from in-patient rehab, I must transition into a new phase: that of outpatient rehab. This means beginning a whole new schedule of therapies in a different building with new people. If you've ever seen the 1991 movie *Regarding Henry*, in which Harrison Ford's character is shot in the head during a botched liquor store holdup and must relearn just about everything, you may recall his remarkable physical therapist, Bradley. This man is the epitome of what a patient needs when going through a recovery period: an always-positive outlook, enthusiasm for every milestone, knowledge of when to push you harder, unflagging belief in your ability. A lot of people underestimate the critical role these therapists play. With their invaluable experience, they not only serve as a coach, but also a quasi-psychotherapist and often a trusted confidant.

When I first meet my therapist, Pauli, she can't believe how well I appear versus how bad my history reads.

"Wow," she says, genuinely surprised, looking me up and down with a huge smile. "You're recovering much faster than I'd expect from the injuries in your chart!"

I'm undeniably proud of myself as I tell her I'm not even sure I need therapy.

She laughs.

I don't blame her. Of course I need further therapy. Who am I kidding?

"I do a lot of visualization," I tell her. "It's been a huge part of my recovery."

I'm not certain how much credence she gives to that in her own therapy protocols, but I'm happy when she tells me, "Whatever you're doing, Ross, it's working, so keep doing it!"

I also tell her that I'm sleeping soundly almost nine hours a night, which is something I've been deprived of for the last six weeks.

"Your body's definitely in repair mode," she says. "It's great that you're getting the sleep you need to facilitate that."

Again, I'm pleased to hear this. I envision that as I get rejuvenating sleep, my muscles are rebuilding and my synapses are reconnecting.

"I must be in overdrive repair mode," I say. "Even with a full night's sleep, I need a few short naps during the day too."

She tells me that makes perfect sense and not to be alarmed. "I'm going to drive you hard in PT. The extra sleep will probably be good for you."

And so begins my three-times-weekly strength, balance, and stamina exercises—all things I can also do at home like grade-school assignments. What's so amazing to me is that *every* muscle group is weakened from my immobility and malnutrition. Pauli works everything from my ankles to my neck. Before now, I didn't even know neck exercises existed. My other therapist, Maureen, is like a drill sergeant, making me do any exercise I struggle with over and over. I treat myself to the same torture when I'm home. *No pain no gain.*

What's frustrating is that I'm making this tremendous progress, but I can't even drive myself to my appointments. In my state, there's a law that if you experience a brain trauma, a physician must sign off on your ability to drive. That's reasonable enough, but if the physician thinks I'm not qualified to drive, I must take a driving course—one offered by *his* hospital and that costs a fair amount of money. Meanwhile, the road is covered with texting teenagers and demented elderly, all of whom are driving without restriction.

The last thing I want is to play this game, or to have word get out that I'm "impaired," so I pay Vasili's gap-year college friend to drive me to physical therapy, telling him I'm simply too weak to drive.

THE PHYSICAL THERAPY makes perfect sense, but I'm surprised when they want to put me through a battery of cognitive exercises as well. I've already done the extensive work of reconnecting my synapses during in-patient rehab; when I speak, it's clear I have no long-lasting issues, yet they still have me labeled as having TBI, or traumatic brain injury.

During my hospitalization, I was in a completely different state. Between the effects of the sedating drugs and the TBI, I had trouble performing certain cognitive tasks. For example, when asked what year it was, I couldn't recall it. It was like being drunk—I felt as if I knew but simply couldn't access it. I could feel myself looking into my brain cortex, asking my cerebral hard drive for the information. I knew what a year was: one rotation of Earth around our solar system's sun; I just didn't know what actual year we were in. In fact, I couldn't even tell you what century we were in. I would have been proud to at least remember 2018, but I was nowhere close. Instead, the number that came to me was 1099. The doctor laughed and told me that was a tax form. Since it was the start of the new year, perhaps that's where my brain went.

"We're actually in the year 2019 now," the doctor said.

Something inside me grasped that she was correct, but I still had the hardest time remembering the precise year, so I set up a mnemonic process to discern it: I could recall 2016 was the last presidential election year and that it was now three years later. Though I wasn't completely confident in my math skills at the time, I could add 16+3 and get 19. Still, because I felt oddly disconnected and couldn't readily pull desired knowledge from wherever it was stored, I wasn't always certain I was correct.

The same random misfiring was evident when they asked me who the current president of the United States was. I could only remember Bill Clinton. Though I knew his term was over, my brain could solely picture blank silhouetted avatars without names after Clinton's final term. In other words, I was aware there were presidents missing, but I couldn't access the names or faces from my brain. A day or two later, Trump materialized in my mind—but Obama was still a nebulous knowledge gap that terrified me. It was like receiving a "file corrupted" message on a laptop—the information was stored somewhere in my neurons, yet I couldn't read the data, despite my desperate search for the proper pathway.

During this time of my confusion while an in-patient, Denise kept my cell phone from me. I wanted it so badly to help pass the time, but she was rightfully concerned that I might text or call someone randomly and reveal the severity of my situation. Being the consummate businessperson, Denise worried about my public image. When she eventually returned my cell phone, she had wiped out my favorites section of telephone numbers so that I wouldn't risk calling someone not in my best interest to contact. But Denise had been one of those favorites, and having her on speed dial meant I rarely had to remember the number. Now, I had the hardest time memorizing it, even after she wrote it down for me. Dementia is like that too: old and routine tasks are easily accomplished because they are hardwired, but new ones are quickly forgotten. Thank goodness they taught me a methodology during my cognitive therapy in in-patient rehab to help me memorize new patterns and information without losing them immediately thereafter. Within a short amount of time, though, even that became unnecessary as my brain returned to completely normal.

The best metaphor I found to describe what I was experiencing with my brain was that of a violently shaken can of yams. Initially, the fibers become mixed with no discernible shape, then, magically over time, the fibers reorganize themselves, like crystallization, back into their original forms. This was how it felt for me as I physically perceived my connections reforming, making details and abilities accessible to my brain. As this occurred, I began thinking in a manner that felt like "the right way" as opposed to my feeling of befuddlement when prompted to answer certain questions.

Within one week of my arrival to in-patient rehab, I was grateful that my new techniques worked for me as quickly as they did and that I was able to recall and give appropriate answers to an untold number of questions. It truly seemed as if a miracle occurred—and perhaps it did. Just like turning on a computer, the neurons began to fire properly, and the connections in my brain became complete, giving me access to the desired data.

Yet now, as an outpatient, it is as if I haven't made this miraculous progress. They ask me to assemble puzzles, solve problems, perform a treasure hunt, all of which I pass with flying colors. Despite this, I'm still considered a patient with TBI, and the physicians on my team assert it will take a very long time to "return to normal." Once again, I resent that I've been given a label, and that this label—rather than my actual ability—puts me on a certain therapeutic road. I understand the outpatient specialists are following what they believe is proper protocol, but I add these disparities to the growing list of things I want to champion when I get back to work.

THE NEXT BIG thing on my list is getting rid of the damn gastrostomy tube. I'm still having issues with my appetite, and I'm convinced this is why. I guess I shouldn't be surprised when the appointment doesn't go as I hope. Not only does the GI doctor not buy my theory, but he wants to do the procedure in a surgical center "just in case."

"If you start to bleed as a result of the tube's removal," he says with gravity, "you should be in a place where we can perform scoping."

As a physician, I know the tube can be easily pulled, and right away see this as a ruse so he can capture a portion of the facility fee.

Denise and I politely turn down his suggestion and leave, opting instead to call the trauma team for an appointment. When we arrive at the trauma center, a medical student under supervision gives the tube a quick yanking motion and out it comes. No bleeding. No complication.

Even better? My appetite returns almost immediately.

The downside is I have a permanent scar on my abdomen that looks like a bullet hole or a second belly button. Coupled with the gladiator scar around my ribcage, and the hollow in my throat from the trach, I look like I've been in a sword fight as well as a gun fight. I don't care so much about the aesthetics except they are a daily reminder of a tragic occurrence. But the feeding tube scar is also a reminder of something else.

Only a few weeks prior to my trauma, a patient came into my office for a consult on a deep abdominal divot above her belly button as a result of having a gastrostomy tube. It reminded her, she told me, of her hospitalization following complications from cancer, and she wanted the scar revised for improvement. At the time, I thought her request self-indulgent, and although I felt I was kind to her, I merely encouraged her to not worry about it. But now, having the exact same defect myself, one I have to feel and look at every day, I see it differently.

My trauma experience has no doubt brought to light numerous improvements the medical profession needs to make in patient care. But as I absorb the regret I now feel for dissuading—and indeed dismissing—this patient's desire to feel more like the woman she was before she was ill, it has also exposed something else: that I myself have been divinely equipped to be an even more empathetic, compassionate physician.

◆

chapter seventeen

ROSS

PICS and PTSD

There is no doubt that I'm healing, but I'm also saddled with an affliction I'd heard of but didn't realize wasn't merely imagined by patients: post-intensive care syndrome, or PICS.

PICS is similar to PTSD—post-traumatic stress disorder—but with traits marked by cognitive, psychiatric, or physical disability after treatment in an intensive care unit. Until now, I had no idea how real or how grave this syndrome is; very few people in the medical profession give it any credence. But I can attest that it's indeed real, and I'm not surprised that the number of patients at risk for it is increasing exponentially as more people survive devastating illness.

My first significant encounter with PICS occurs during my initial week at home when I crawl into bed each night. The bed itself feels heavenly—but the covers trigger claustrophobic anxiety. Though it is winter, I cannot tolerate the heavy comforter over my body; even the tight feeling of sheets over my feet seems so restricting that I feel as if I'm in a coffin. After sleeping in hospital beds for six weeks straight with only a thin sheet or blanket on top of me, the only way I can sleep with any ease is to toss the bedding off me completely.

I also have trouble getting out of bed—and not just because I'm dealing with weakness that makes it a strain on my core to sit up, needing to cheat by using my arms instead of my abdominal muscles to push myself upright. Each time I go to get up, flashes from the "brainwashing" that I wasn't allowed to get up on my own, and how militant the nurses could be about keeping us confined in our beds, feels like an invisible control taking hold of me. I crave the autonomy of getting up as I please, yet when I do, I feel a blast of fear. I relate it to a heavily disciplined child being on his own for the first time at camp, having a blissful sense of freedom, yet sensing an ever-present parental eye always watching and waiting for him to make a wrong move worthy of punishment.

I'm further affected by PICS through an irrational fear I find myself coming back to daily. Though I'm the luckiest person in the world, with minimal physical problems from the fall, I can't help but obsess over the fact that had I landed an inch to the right or left, I could have severed my spine or crushed my head. While I'm incredibly grateful that didn't actually occur, I consistently worry that what *didn't* happen during the fall will somehow come to fruition *now*. In other words, I have this illogical concern that my recovery period will evolve for the *worse*, not the better. Every time I forget something, I think, *Could it be an exacerbation of my brain injury?* One of my favorite novels I read in high school was *Flowers for Algernon*, where the protagonist, Charlie Gordon, has a developmental delay and is successfully given a test vaccine to increase his intelligence. The tragedy is that as the effect of the vaccine wears off, he is painfully aware of his mental decline. In a similar vein, I wonder, *What if I suddenly turn less bright?* Sotiri had told everyone in the ICU that even if I was mentally damaged by half, I would still be smarter than everyone in the room. His sentiment was heartwarming, but it was true that my brain had gotten me to where I am. The notion that I could be slated for a similar fate as Charlie threatened to paralyze me. Luckily, I fought hard against it. But I could see how for some people, such a belief could indeed be crippling.

My facial paralysis is a stark reminder of the ICU too. I have always been able to wink only with my left eye, and when my face was paralyzed from the temporal bone fracture, it was my left facial nerve that no longer fired. I distinctly remember the physical therapists walking me back and forth in the step-down unit, and me trying desperately to wink at Denise as we passed her. I sent the signals from my brain, but nothing happened. I can only imagine what it looked like to my wife: a monster with a drooping face. The nerve is fully functioning again now, thank God, but winking at Denise never fails to bring me back to when it didn't.

Even something as basic as my fingers hurl me back into the depths of my trauma. I don't recall having horizontal grooves in my nails, especially not all of them. But I do now—and they've become more apparent as they've grown out. Like tree rings in a stump, nails will become marked during times of trauma. When I consider the rate of nail growth, these grooves clearly started as a result of severe malnutrition while I was in the hospital. Every time I begin to mindlessly rub these grooves, I'm right back in the ICU again. I know they'll grow out with time, but for now they still serve as a daily reminder.

And I'm not the only one afflicted by symptoms of PICS. Those who stay with a patient in the ICU are just as susceptible to the psychologic strains; worrying about whether a loved one will survive or how bills will be paid takes an enormous toll. After being traumatized by witnessing my oxygen saturation fall and my needing to be intubated multiple times during my

ICU stay, Denise lies awake at night, carefully listening to my breathing, feeling responsible to monitor if I suddenly breathe irregularly. If I do, she awakens me and asks if I'm okay. When she does sleep soundly for a period of time, she is startled upon waking, hopeful she hasn't "let" anything happen to me in the night. She likewise has a fear reaction every time I call her, scared that I may be in potential danger. Even if she's in a work meeting, she jumps up and leaves so she can immediately take my call.

PICS is also fickle: it can affect two people very differently, depending on the trigger. For instance, in an attempt to help me feel normal, Denise brought one of my t-shirts to the step-down unit for me to wear during my first ambulance transfer to the rehab facility. I had not yet been decannulated, so my tracheostomy tube jutted out of my neck and the shirt couldn't lie right at the throat. I asked the nurse to cut the neck vertically with scissors along the midline; after making it a V-neck, the shirt no longer interfered with the tube. At some point, Denise wanted to throw that shirt out, but I wouldn't let her. I saw it as a victory: I was decannulated, I survived. For me, that shirt became a symbol of my strength as well as a reminder of the need for good luck, whereas for Denise, the altered shirt is nothing but a painful reminder.

Although research exists that supports minimizing sedation and promoting early mobilization to decrease the risk of developing PICS, few healthcare providers really know about this syndrome—and even fewer are trying to prevent it. Lucky for me, without knowing PICS was a problem we wanted to avoid, Denise championed my getting off the narcotics and into physical rehab as soon as possible. In my opinion, this is the main reason, along with all the prayers people said for me, that I'm able to be home so soon.

I WISH I could say that PICS is the only psychological syndrome I'm managing, but the truth is, I am haunted by a form of PTSD as well. Similar to a returning veteran, multiple sights, sounds, and events trigger feelings of unease in me, or catapult me to another time or place in my mind, that take time to settle down.

For example, immediately after my return home, I am irrationally fearful that I may die as a complication of my trauma. Clearly, this is not going to happen, but I'm plagued with negative thoughts nonetheless.

What if I develop fatal pneumonia because I'm not breathing as deeply as I should due to the hardware? The use of thoracic plates is relatively new and there is very little long-term follow-up data. When I caught my first cold shortly after coming home, I was constantly checking my sputum to inspect for the difference between post-nasal drip and lung infection.

What if I'm in another accident and something fiercely hits my chest plates? I'm so paranoid that I find myself covering this part of my chest when someone merely comes too close to me.

What if my heart stops and the attempts to perform cardiopulmonary resuscitation fail due to the rigidity of the plates, preventing appropriate chest compressions?

When I'm in the shower, I feel as if I went to sleep and awoke with a different body. All of the bumps and lines from my new scars are startling every time I see and feel them: substantial divots on my chest from the chest tubes; keloids that dot my radial wrist from multiple arterial line placements; scars on the inner sides of my elbows from the hundreds of blood draws. Incisions from the plating, drains, gastrostomy tube, and tracheostomy are now closed but the skin is tight.

New lumps pop up too, like the one on my lateral thorax.

When I press downward, I feel a collection of muscle fibers that weren't placed back into their native location; during the thoracotomy, a portion of my serratus muscle along the rib cage was not meticulously repaired. While this doesn't affect my physiology in any way, it is one of numerous physical symbols of the price I paid to survive.

And there's more.

When water gets into my ears, the muffled sound instantly takes me to when my ears were filled with blood. On the left side of my chest the skin is numb, so hugging is less enjoyable. When I carry things pressed against that side, the absent sensation serves as an active reminder of what happened to me. All the swelling and immobility I've suffered has created internal scar bands that limit my range and strength. This is something I see frequently in my abdominoplasty patients, and now I'm experiencing it firsthand. I often feel as if I'm wearing a tight straitjacket and someone has wrapped his hands around my throat. I know it will take months, maybe years, for the tightness and redness of the scars to fade, but they will never vanish or stop serving to be a harsh reminder. I may not have gotten my wounds sacrificing for my country, but I did emerge from a personal battle, one that has given me a heightened appreciation for our military every time the fireworks of scars splayed across my body stare back at me.

And the tones of certain beeps, buzzes, and hums? They propel me right back into that ICU bed where I felt so isolated, frustrated, and confined.

It's tough on Denise as well. She is haunted by images of me on the ground every time she pulls into our driveway or looks out the window on that side of the house. She can barely stand to see anything that resembles a tube or a wire after seeing me hooked up to so many for so long. And she, too, can't seem to shake the terror certain beeps and sounds bring forth.

There are, however, two triggers that have two sides to them: a stressor *and* a blessing.

Right before my fall, Denise gave me an early Christmas gift I could start using for our holiday celebrations: a freezer tray that makes round ice balls for drinks. The day before the accident, I made and stored a supply in a Ziploc baggie. Simply finding them in the freezer made Denise break down; she couldn't bear to use them and hid them behind other items in the freezer drawer. When I uncovered them after my return home, all I could think was how innocent I was when I last touched them. They were a stark reminder that I was blessed by surviving my trauma—and also supremely aware of how ephemeral life can be. Had I died, despite the seeming lack of substance those ice cubes held, I know it would have destroyed Denise to let them melt away.

The other trigger comes from the feathers released that afternoon when EMS cut open my down vest to resuscitate me. Still suspended in the cobwebs of our garage, they mockingly remind us both of the trauma—and by extension the random nature of our existence. Each feather now serves as a *memento mori*, a Latin phrase meaning "remember that you will die." This may sound morbid, but I view it as a reminder of the transient nature of life, that the ephemerality and delicate nature of our existence must never be forgotten, that the only thing that matters is what we create, not what we accumulate. In other words, our creations, whatever they may be, should reflect our character so that we can be a better person and thereby make the world a better place. While Denise would prefer these feathers cleaned away, I find satisfaction—even meaning—in how they hover almost like angels, serving a beneficial role in our lives.

It is one thing to intellectually believe we should live each day as if it could be our last, but it is completely different to emotionally understand its significance.

◆

chapter eighteen

ROSS

Reunion

Only two weeks after my discharge from the rehabilitation hospital, I don my finest shirt, blazer, and shoes to visit the ICU at the trauma hospital. Though I feel somewhat weak, and I must cinch my belt to the last hole to keep my ill-fitting pants up, I'm strong enough to walk and talk. Even more gratifying is that not one person recognizes me.

The shriveled, skinny, non-verbal old man with a tracheostomy, arterial line, gastrostomy tube, and gray facial hair is gone; the man they see has morphed into a relatively normal adult—so much so that it is only when the nurses recognize Denise that they subsequently realize who I am.

"Ross!" one physician assistant blurts out. "Look at you!"

I smile. I feel overwhelming gratitude for how far I've come in the four weeks since they've seen me. Despite the lingering trauma from my time here, it is my dream come true to thank everyone for their hard work that saved my life.

"For you," I say to my trauma surgeon, handing him a bottle of my favorite bourbon. "I can't thank you enough for everything you did for me."

He pats me gently on the back. "It was my pleasure."

We take celebratory photographs. We exchange jubilant

hugs. Nurse after nurse is amazed to see me. One, who had been on duty when I climbed out of bed and fell as a result, begins to cry, seemingly grateful that everything turned out all right.

Most shocking, though, is the reaction of the ICU medical director—the physician who had erroneously told my family that it would likely take many months to a year for me to return to normal, if that was even possible. Now I stand before him, just shy of two months after my trauma. It is an understatement to say that he is nonplussed.

I had lain in my ICU bed vowing I would return to this same unit as a human being, and there are no words to describe how it feels to achieve that goal.

Yet, I feel as if I harbor a great secret.

I may appear intact and healthy on the outside; anyone seeing me walk the hallways of the hospital that day would think I'm visiting a sick relative, not celebrating my own recovery. But on a level no one around me can understand, I am visiting myself. Through dogged perseverance and a smidgeon of luck, I set a goal and achieved it. Now, standing on the other side of the glass, staring at the same ICU bay that held me, I picture my withered body hooked up to the ventilator and decide I cannot bury that version of Ross. I need to hold on to him and grow from his experience. He is part of my new lexicon, of the story those who encounter me don't know. This is true for everyone, that we rarely know of the personal trials people have faced. Not one living person escapes suffering; we must remember this dictum always. It is the Stoic process of accepting this fate, even loving it, that makes us stronger.

Against the din of the excitement, I smile internally at the picture of ICU Ross in my mind's eye—another *memento mori* —and know beyond a shadow of a doubt that my memory of him ensures two things: compassion and empathy for my patients will forever be my guiding light as a physician; and I will use my experience to do everything in my power to vastly improve the field of medicine.

◆

chapter nineteen

ROSS
Return

When I entered the rehab facility on January 25, 2019, my physicians targeted June as my earliest return date to the office, and months longer before I would operate again. But I had eschewed those predictions and declared to Denise that I would be back to work in only four weeks. I knew she might be skeptical, but she maintained her utmost faith in me as I told her how I was persistently visualizing myself in my office, engaging with patients, and returning to the operating room. Despite the challenges, I never believed I wouldn't fulfill my goal.

Two months after my trauma, I return to my office, just as I imagined.

I have some residual weakness in my shoulders, but I continue to perform daily exercises to improve my range. I thank God that my surgical specialty is known for delicate work and not brute force. One of the biggest parts of my recovery has come from having a procedure called myofascial scar release. Release of this tissue involves a suction machine that cups the skin off the underlying muscle while a therapist stretches the tissues. This results in pulling the scar and releasing the internal scar bands. If you imagine this hurts, you're right. But my therapist, MaryEllen, does a remarkable job, and after the treatment, the skin is not only much more pliable, but my range has dramatically improved. The soreness lasts for days, but it is well worth it. In fact, Denise and I purchase a cupping machine so I can continue these treatments at home.

I am not a magician, nor superhuman, but I am a testament to what laser focus on survival and recovery can look like. I have no doubt that my visualization exercises played a tremendous role in my journey toward wholeness. The mind-body connection is irrefutable. I also cannot discount the tremendous number of prayers I've received without my knowing it. Each time I'm in a hospital working as a physician, staff members tell me they were praying for me. I am overwhelmed by their caring and am grateful beyond words. I have no doubt that all the positive energy from these colleagues and strangers contributed to my successful recovery.

My thoughts once again return to what it must be like for returning veterans as I wonder what I've done to deserve such a favorable outcome.

Shortly after resuming direct patient care, I am back to performing surgeries.

I'M FULLY AWARE of what I'm currently capable of, and I would never put a patient at risk of not receiving my best surgical ability, but it is no surprise that not everyone in my circle believes I'm ready to perform surgeries. Once again, I prove them wrong. I'm keeping my schedule less demanding so that I'm well rested, and I have aches in parts of my body—which are exacerbated by increased humidity, as I've heard people say for years. But thankfully, the limitations quickly fade.

The truth is, I am a better physician now than I was before my fall. I spend more time talking to patients and getting to know them. In fact, I no longer allow my staff to double book patients in the office. I always loved medicine, but now I want to touch people's lives in a more personal way. I find I also bond much more rapidly with my patients because it's one thing to explain a complex surgery and its recovery, but it is entirely another to experience it personally. Doctors tend to rush because there is so much to do: obtaining the history, performing the examination, creating a list of possible diagnoses and mapping a care plan. Documentation has taken on a crushing role, and electronic records take time to navigate and complete—not to mention doctors get paid based on seeing patients, so time is of the essence.

But my experiences have made me reconsider everything. I want to connect more with patients regardless of the financial consequences to me. One of my mentor surgeons in Iowa, Dr. Brian McCabe, always asked his residents in lectures, "Just how much is enough money to make?" It was then that I realized people should certainly satisfy their personal financial wellness, but not fall for the treadmill of accumulation. Yes, I now earn less money each day, but spending extra time with each patient brings me far greater reward than money ever could. It's also a reflection of the Stoic value of subtraction: since we must realize life is short, what is behind the purpose of mere accumulation?

As a plastic surgeon, I have a significant role to play in the lives of those who need what I've been trained to offer. One manifestation of this is that I frequently manage patients who were involved in life-altering trauma that severed their spinal cord and resulted in permanent paralysis, which often leads to pressure sores. One such patient, about my age, had metal rods holding him together and had acquired a pressure sore as a result of sitting unrelieved too long in his wheelchair. As I interviewed him and his wife, something deep in my brain screamed out to me how lucky I was. *By the grace of God, there go I.*

Another patient with a pressure sore had to postpone his surgery with me while I was recovering. When I was able to reschedule the procedure, he asked how I was doing. Looking at him, lying on a gurney, paralyzed from the waist down, I saw a brother-in-arms. Humbly, I said, "I'm the luckiest person in the world."

"You certainly are," his wife acknowledged. She pointed to her spouse with a pained face. "You could be where he is."

Every time I see someone with traumatic paralysis, I feel immense empathy for them, and immense gratitude for myself. I am constantly aware that I've been granted an inexplicable gift not to be in a wheelchair—and how easily it could have been different.

When I take paralyzed patients to the operating room to clean infected wounds, I stand guard over them. As we position patients carefully on the operating table, I'm no longer solely focused on perfectionistic details, but rather see a vulnerable person who didn't ask for this misfortune and who has placed complete trust in me. Where I previously felt a fiduciary duty to protect these patients, I now connect with them deeply on an emotional level.

I'm also acutely aware of the plight of the spouses. When they married their beloved, they never imagined he or she would become paralyzed. Denise never made me feel like a burden, and she didn't have to help me perform banal tasks for very long. But for these people, it is their new everyday reality. I sympathize with how emotionally draining it is for them, how tired these people must be helping their partners get out of bed, get dressed, use the bathroom. I have a newfound understanding of how traumatic it is for them to witness their loved one struggle with self-care and self-confidence. Whereas I used to see the spouses as a more peripheral presence, I now see them as people who desperately need support too.

ANOTHER GIFT I'VE received since being back to work is being touched by how my established patients have been so concerned about my health. Those who were rescheduled to allow me to recover show genuine sympathy. At the end of a consultation, when I as the physician would typically place a hand on the patient's shoulder for reassurance, many of my patients now place their hand on *my* shoulder, or even hug me. I also find we often share a kinship, one that only those who go through these types of major life events personally understand. People who have survived as we have know firsthand the silent battles required to win the overall war—the journey it requires, the toll it takes. We fight these battles daily while the average person erroneously believes all is well with us, because we may look it on the outside. Those who haven't experienced such an event are ignorant of this part of recovery, but we as victors know how to drink in the daily miracles of life: the majesty of the blue sky, the life-giving oxygen of the trees, the unconditional love of a spouse, the list goes on. Each of these gifts of grace brings serenity to what could be an otherwise tumultuous daily routine.

One of my patients, who received a kidney transplant from his own wife, expresses heartfelt empathy for what I go through on a day-to-day basis, seeming to understand me on a fundamental level. Every time I see him, he asks how I feel.

Recently, I performed a procedure on him, and when the nurses asked him if he needed help with his gown to protect his modesty, he laughed.

"As the doc knows," he said, "modesty is no longer an issue after what we've been through."

This simple acknowledgment of my situation was touching. At times, it actually feels as if my patients are doctoring me.

It also hasn't taken long for me to discover the number of people who know someone who died after falling from a height. One operating-room nurse told me how her father, who was a fireman, died after falling while working on his own home. Tragically, her brother-in-law had a similar accident and died as well. A physician who works in one of the hospitals I attend told me how his mother-in-law fell while working on her roof and subsequently died. All of these robust people suffered an unexpected mishap the same way I did, but none of them survived. Over and over again, I cannot believe my luck.

A FEW WEEKS after my return to the OR, I am headed down the hospital stairwell when I see an in-patient with a cane struggling to go up the stairs, with his physical therapist coaching him. I stop dead in my tracks. How far I've come and how lucky I am strike me like lightning.

"Excuse me," I say, stopping them. "I just wanted you to know that only three months ago, I was in your exact situation." I loosen my tie and show him my tracheostomy scar. His eyes widen. "The best advice I can give you is to visualize your success," I tell him. "Work hard on your recovery and never give up. I have no doubt you can do it."

He tears up and thanks me.

Overwhelmed by gratitude and how fragile life is, I mirror his emotion and cry too.

And that female patient I had deferred surgery for only a

few months prior? I call and invite her back to my office, apologizing for not having more understanding at the time and explaining what happened to me. "I'll be more than happy to revise your gastrostomy scar," I tell her.

A few weeks later, she gives me that second chance. As I perform the procedure, I observe with fascination the scar bands leading from the skin to the deep fascia. These are the same bands responsible for my similar pains and the divot in my skin. But most gratifying is her reaction when she comes in for her follow-up.

She couldn't be more pleased with the result.

And I couldn't be more humbled to witness it.

◆

chapter twenty

ROSS

Aftermath

In the well-known Kübler-Ross model of grief, she outlines five stages people travel through: denial, anger, bargaining, depression, and acceptance. I admit I had always been skeptical of psychology, but I can attest that these stages are real. While Denise touched on her experiences with this in Chapter Six, my true awareness and understanding was delayed, making my journey different.

In the denial stage, I persistently told Denise I was ready to leave the hospital. I clearly had no rationale for how I would breathe, how Denise would suction out my tracheostomy, how I would strengthen my limbs without aggressive physical therapy. I erroneously believed that as a physician, I'd somehow manage.

When I transitioned into anger, I would lie in the hospital—when I was coherent enough to think—and ponder, *Why did this happen to me? I've dedicated myself to being a surgeon . . . this is completely unfair. I even volunteer in Guatemala on a yearly basis, and now I must miss my annual trip. How is that even right?* I recognized that these feelings were juvenile and decided not to share them with anyone, but they plagued me nonetheless.

In short order, I landed in the minefield of bargaining. *If only I could leave the hospital soon, I'd rejoin the medical staff of this trauma hospital where I previously worked and treat indigent patients for free. If only I could be without any physical or mental consequences from this fall, I'd become more religious. Because I'm alive, I'll dedicate more of my energy to listening to my patients. I will never be short again if only I emerge from this unscathed.* I also allowed chaplains to come into my room and pray for me, regardless of their religion. I suppose I decided to play the numbers, just in case.

Once I returned home, I rapidly moved on to acceptance, thinking I'd skipped depression altogether. Whenever I encountered someone who showed me sympathy, I'd say, "All's well that ends well." And since I *was* doing remarkably well, I completely accepted everything. "No harm no foul" became a sort of mantra. I reasoned that all the pain and suffering no longer mattered because there were minimal long-term consequences. My spine and brain were intact, which was a lot more than many victims of a fall like mine could say. My Stoic philosophy had me believing it was futile to fight what I couldn't control.

But then the murky feeling of depression sneaked up on Denise and me. It was never so bad that either of us contemplated medication. Nevertheless, I did find myself glum at times and didn't feel quite myself. What I desired deeply was to talk to people who had experienced similar trauma, but there was nowhere to go; no local or even regional support group existed for people who survived crazy falls and ICU stays. I also realized I was somewhat down perhaps because it became glaringly real that life can change in an instant. In the second it takes to simply snap our fingers, everything we know can be drastically altered. We realize this in theory, but we rarely acknowledge or even experience it. My massive chest wall scar is a daily reminder, one that initially caused overwhelming sadness in me each time I saw it, that everything I'd built could instantly disappear. Sometimes it truly felt like luck played a critical role and there was little we could control. But then I'd replay what might have happened on the roof that day and consider if I could have prevented my fall or if the outcome could have been much worse. All these thoughts led me to wonder if the depression people commonly experience following brain injury is not merely part of the neurologic recovery, but rather a coming to grips with the fickle nature of life.

Decades ago—and still today in developing countries—people were regularly faced with numerous harsh realities: women perishing in childbirth; children dying of illness; marauders descending unannounced upon villages and killing randomly; the list goes on. In the developed world, because these events are so infrequent, when they do occur, our society's reaction is chaotic. Living in a bubble, we forget—or even ignore—the fragility of our existence. The ancients knew well how brittle existence could be, as the original Greek acolytes of Stoicism were indeed slaves to the Romans. Hence, in my opinion, for us to consistently make meaning of our relatively short lives, we must embrace constructive values and strive to live them daily.

Having experienced every stage of grief, what I knew was this: I had two choices. I could remain a victim who was angry at the world for screwing with me, or I could recognize the majesty of my luck. I chose the latter, and that's what I've held fast to ever since.

WHILE I'VE UNDOUBTEDLY elected to walk on the sunny side of the street from here forward, I can't ignore that everyday activities serve as reminders of my trauma. Ironically, the severity of it doesn't lie in the actual fall from the roof, but rather the multitude of interventions the physicians employed to keep me alive.

For example, I have no problem climbing up ladders or standing at a height; I've already resumed changing burned-out lightbulbs and batteries in our smoke detectors. But when I turn my head in a certain direction, I feel the skin pull at my throat from the tracheostomy scar. When I talk, I can no longer speak in long sentences because my lung capacity is diminished from the rib plating. I find myself having to repeat things to cashiers in noisy places because I can't project in a strong voice.

And, for a period of time, another reminder haunted me too.

In the backyard using the grill one day, I looked up and saw the caulking gun and old caulk tube lying beside the metal frame of the skylight, exactly where I left them when I went to get more material that December day. A sickening feeling swept over me. Those were the last things I touched before my life irrevocably changed. These simple tools were a physical marker of my transition. Like the feathers, they were a *memento mori*. I thought perhaps I should see the positive aspect of this event and leave them in place. But I realized in that moment that I couldn't, as these were *my* tokens, not my family's.

A few months later—nearly six months to the day of my fall—we had our gutters cleaned. I asked the professionals (who I noted were wearing helmets, something that never occurred to me to do while working on my house) if they would get my supplies off the roof. When they handed them to me, I felt a wave of depression come over me. These items, symbolic of the dividing line between innocence and near death, were now in my hands. These were no longer *memento mori*, but rather just regular household items. Their power was gone. My somber reaction clearly confounded the workers; to them, they were just basic home-improvement necessities.

I startled them by pulling up my shirt. "These are my scars from falling off the roof the day I was using these supplies," I say. "I'm sure I don't have to remind you guys to be extra careful in your job."

Their eyes grew wide and they asked me to share more of my story.

As I volunteered the details, I hoped that hearing my cautionary tale would save them from possibly having a tragic accident themselves.

I also feel strong resistance to tempting fate, as though I've already used up my "nine lives" to survive the fall. When I pull my car into the garage, I stare longingly at my motorcycle. *Would it be irresponsible of me to ride it again?* I wonder. *How could I possibly risk doing something reckless again? If I were to have an accident, would it be worse now because I have metal plates in my chest? Would my chest crumble more easily now that there are healed fractures? Would God say I was a complete idiot for riding my motorcycle, and I therefore forfeited my chance to live longer on his Earth?*

Even taking a simple bicycle ride during a family outing following my return home made me feel somewhat reticent. *What if I fall or am unsteady and ride into traffic?* I thought. *I haven't gained all my strength back yet.* But I refused to show my unease. I knew my injury had negatively impacted my loved ones and didn't want to make it worse for them. As it was, three pairs of prying eyes checked on me frequently as I struggled through the physically grueling ride. While I'm certainly not handicapped, I'm treated as fragile at times—which is at once a loving gesture and sometimes difficult to swallow as a grown man.

But despite these apparent stumbling blocks, I saw a grand opportunity before me after fortune granted my second chance. Besides altering my practice to better suit my goals of helping people, I was determined to improve my physical health. I gained back only fifteen of the thirty pounds I lost, the vast percentage of which was muscle, not fat. As a result, my blood pressure is better controlled, and my blood sugars run less high.

I also vowed to appreciate every moment, relating profoundly to the character of Emily in Thornton Wilder's *Our Town*. After dying tragically while giving birth to her second child, she is granted the ability to travel back in time and view a segment of her life. As she watches her parents interact, she asks to return to the cemetery, proclaiming, "Living people don't understand!" These simple words express that she is gravely disappointed by how humans don't appreciate their time on this earth. I don't want to be one of those people.

Because I treasure life so much more than I did before, I also have a heightened awareness of what it means to be careful. I now drive more purposefully, and I ask Denise to be extra cautious, particularly in the kitchen. When she's preparing food, for example, I easily conjure the image of the knife slipping from her hand and slicing her or cutting off a finger. My brain never did that before, but it seems to not be able to help itself now.

I find, too, that Denise and I both pay more attention to the news when an individual needlessly dies; death from an accident seems so tragic. We not only relive our own pain each time, but we also deeply feel the pain and grief of the victim's family like never before. It is one thing to sympathize with the suffering of another, but now we're truly able to empathize, which takes compassion to a whole new level.

I HAVE ALSO been profoundly reflective on the subject of human nature, compelled to analyze certain people's actions, over the timeline of my trauma. In doing so, I've observed both the bright and the dim sides, in a multitude of ways.

First, why did an EMT cut my favorite down vest when he could have easily just unzipped it? I know the paramedics needed to inspect me quickly, but using scissors to do so was unnecessary. However, while I would suggest rethinking that protocol, I am also moved by the fact that this person provided me with a lifelong metaphor for the tenuousness of existence—as well as with the title of this book.

Why did our new neighbor, whom we hadn't even met, zigzag around police cars and two ambulances to watch emergency paramedics work on me? I was bloody and sprawled on the driveway, and Denise was hysterical, yet at the exact moment the paramedics were prepping me for transport, she introduced herself. A human being was clearly injured and his spouse was obviously devastated. What was she thinking? After she satisfied her curiosity, she left. No subsequent well wishes. No note or food dropped off afterward. I decided I was lucky she didn't film the scene with her phone and post it on YouTube or Facebook. Too many people have become vicarious thrill seekers, viewing tragic events solely as a means of entertainment, perhaps as a result of watching hours of YouTube without any moral code. I can't help but wonder, with all the disasters now captured on cell phone video, if we have lost our humanity in our growing detachment from cataclysmic events. I still occasionally Google "people falling off roof" to make sure there are no surreptitious videos of my trauma on the Internet.

In observing my family, I have deep conflict too. My father was extraordinarily helpful when I was incapacitated in the ICU. He was professorial in helping Denise with some complex medical decisions, and he voluntarily managed quite a few of my patients. But, as I've already shared, my parents also disappointed me with their coldness and distance. Beyond that, they chose not to inform any of my non-nuclear relatives about my trauma. Was it mentally easier for them not to rehash all the details? Did they prefer to ignore the severity of my injuries, or perhaps avoid the barrage of phone calls and questions? No matter their reasoning, I believe such decisions should be made with respect to what is best for the patient. When I was in rehabilitation, I had no other visitors but my immediate family. When I was home recuperating, none of my cousins, aunts, or uncles called to support me when I needed them the most because they didn't even know what had happened to me. As Denise was, thankfully, laser-focused on me at that time, she wasn't thinking about distant family members she only saw infrequently, so she didn't contact them either. (As an amusing side note: although I'd briefly lamented these people not being part of my support circle, it made for laughable conversations when I called to let relatives know I had nearly died two months previously. Even those who had recently spoken to my folks were still unaware.)

My father's storming out of my hospital room and ceasing to speak to me after I simply asked for my CT scans to be returned—which he had requested to analyze—is something I surmised as a grudge that he wasn't "in charge." I understand how the stress of a severely injured son can devastate a parent, but the focus should always be doing the right thing. In a situation such as mine involving the brain, family members must think of those involved as if in a military hierarchy: the patient is the general, and the next in command is his or her spouse serving as the power of attorney (POA). In other words, when a patient is debilitated, the POA is in charge. In our case, that was Denise, which meant it was incumbent upon my parents to recognize they were not in control and shouldn't entertain that notion.

This arrangement can cause tension in families at a time of illness, as the spouse may not hold the same view regarding financial or business decisions as the parents. This is what occurred when my father was unable to be in charge the way he wanted, generating severe dysfunction in my recovery that could easily have been avoided. In other words, when the patient (the general in this metaphor) returns, power (or command) must be returned without issue.

Even actions taken by my brother, which were supposedly rooted in love and concern, were unintentionally damaging. During my ICU stay, Brett contacted a friend who was a medical chief of an ICU in a prestigious hospital. My brother fed him information about my case, and the colleague mechanically agreed that my recovery would at best take many months. This compounded Denise's terror by hindering her unbridled optimism. How can a doctor give an opinion when he's never physically examined the patient? How can he assume the facts given by a family member were accurate? Yet the doctor proclaimed a diagnosis remotely and my family blindly accepted this as truth—a "truth" they felt compelled to repeatedly remind my wife and me as they watched us pour what they thought was futile hope into my ability to quickly recover.

I have great disappointment, too, in the plastic surgeon to whom my staff electively referred many of my patients while I was in the hospital. I mistook him to be a collegial friend, yet shortly after my return to work, he told me during a telephone call that I initiated to thank him for his help just how "jealous" he was of my practice. In fact, he subsequently pursued a position at one of the hospitals where I formerly attended, so blinded by jealousy that he rushed to be paid by the very hospital that received a D grade from the Leapfrog Group. There could be no better example of how uncapped emotion can destroy an individual. If I were asked to help an ill colleague, I would never think of trying to replace him; in fact, I would encourage the patients who could wait to hold off until the injured surgeon returned. In my case, however, this surgeon did not actively tell my patients of my recovery; my office had to inform these patients that I returned. I realize that this lack of true collegiality amongst competing doctors is likely a result of the fact that doctors are reimbursed based on volume—and that pits physicians against each other. While this is deplorable, I vow to maintain my core principles of helping patients, knowing I can influence by example, but not control the actions of others.

Sadly, my relationship with this colleague wasn't the only one that proved disappointing; several turned out to be disingenuous. Their texts to me and offers to Denise saying they wanted to celebrate with me after I got better were only empty words. After I returned home, few bothered to take the time or energy to get together. The friends who did were truly special.

Applying Stoic philosophy, I acknowledge that most people are motivated by selfish behavior, but I likewise see my lesson in these people's actions: never make empty promises to people.

When you are truly ill, you hear many empty promises and

wishes offered out of obligation, but the truth is that many people don't actually follow through. While this brought me down at first, I was grateful to quickly come back to the Stoic belief that anger is the enemy of logic, creating strife that need not exist, and that it is personally destructive and serves no purpose. I am aware that anger rots the core, like cancer, so I am not angry at these people; I realize I cannot control their actions, only my reaction to their actions. As Seneca (the Stoic who served as Nero's counselor two thousand years ago) explains, how does getting even at a dog that bites me by biting him back serve any purpose?

I had to remember this aphorism when the hospital where I was seriously concerned about plummeting quality and filed multiple reports regarding lapses in safety put me on a one-year leave of absence after my injury, rather than simply approving my removal from the on-call schedule as two other hospitals had. In fact, I was quickly terminated as the medical director of two service lines, ignoring my written contract, which states a termination must be in writing. Instead, while I was in the ICU, I received word through the grapevine that my leadership in these positions was no longer required. That was it. No thank you. No acknowledgment while I lay intubated and nearly dead of how I grew these services. I had received a stipend for these positions, and the hospital administrators found the opportunity they had been looking for to save money: they could now divert the funds away from me and direct them instead to a physician group whom they desperately wanted to keep at the hospital for the referrals. It didn't matter that I had built these well-recognized service lines and successfully maintained quality for over 15 years. Manipulating my tragedy for the hospital's financial gain was pathetic, and linking my firing to my decreasing volume was arguably illegal. But I had just lived through a near-death trauma, and as a result, I no longer felt the need to sweat these kinds of things, no matter how egregious the behavior. I knew deep down those involved in these maneuvers were barreling toward leaving a less-than-favorable legacy, while I was being guided toward something more aligned with my values.

Although I observed several disheartening actions along the timeline of my trauma and recovery period, with every drop in my faith in humanity, I was buoyed tenfold. I received dozens and dozens of meaningful letters, notes, and small gifts from many patients and some of my close colleagues, all of which were both touching and meaningful. To be the focus of such an outpouring of love was amazing. The irony of wishing a healer that he heals well was not lost on me; I saved each one of those notes and reread them often during my recovery. Even seemingly minor gestures were clearly full of love and sincerely appreciated, such as when one of Denise's close work friends dropped off a hot lunch while Denise stood vigil for me in the ICU. This is the kind of action I will never forget.

Furthermore, I do not underestimate the power of prayer. So many patients and nurses told me that they prayed for my recovery. While I don't pretend to understand how it all works, I cannot help but think there is a strong connection to my speedy and complete recovery. I was deeply moved that I had positively affected so many peoples' lives such that when I needed prayers, there were plenty of people there for me. Although an angel must have protected me during my fall when I hit the ground, it was this love through prayer that somehow managed to sustain me afterward.

But perhaps the true brass ring I've grabbed is what I refer to as "my new superpower."

Comic books nicely illustrate some important Stoic principles. Nearly every superhero experiences a traumatic event that grants a new power. He or she is then faced with the dilemma of how to use this gift. Though Denise thought I was crazy, I became determined to uncover my superpower, to unleash a silver lining in the cloud of my trauma.

After very little thought, my superpower came to me: Clarity of Vision. In other words, I now possess the ability to ignore true crap. This means I no longer care about things outside my sphere of control, and I can laugh off the petty actions of others. It is as if the Stoic mantras floating in my head at the time of my fall were magically seared into the synapses of my brain, making me a living, breathing super-being.

This Clarity of Vision helps me realize what I can and cannot control, or rather, the futility of "tilting at windmills." This notion comes from the well-known literary character, Don Quixote, who proves the inability of a single person to fight the forces of evil, no matter how chivalrous the effort. I realize that although I have the power to change injustice, striving to do it alone only makes me a martyr. For example, whereas I wasted so much energy before my trauma trying to achieve the impossible by changing the quality of a hospital, I now think, *Why not just stop operating there? Why bring a patient to a facility that earns Cs and most recently a D, where patients have a statistically greater chance of dying from an error? Why not only attend hospitals that place the patient first and earn an A? Moreover, if I help educate people about these measures, I can help even those who are not my patients.* This simple action better reflects my values and allows me to avoid unnecessary battles.

Further, Denise has noticed I'm much more tranquil than before the trauma. My office staff has said the same. I still want to get things accomplished and finish jobs both in a timely fashion and with an outstanding quality of care, but the smaller things don't bother me as they used to. How can I get upset about something minor when it is a gift to simply be alive on this planet?

My superpower also enables me to make my practice what I want it to be, not caring about what other physicians may think about my passion (if not zeal) for patient quality. Those who understand and agree with me will follow suit; those who feel threatened by it may try to defame me. My response to that is: *So what.* That's the beauty of my new superpower.

And there's more.

Every time I pull into my driveway, I see the dent in the gutter over the garage and think how it is a blessing to remain with the person I love most, my wife. I am grateful to live constructively. I know what is required of true friendship and unconditional love, and I know how to honor receiving it by reflecting it back. I'm devoted to cherishing everything, to celebrating the here and now of life, because it simply does not last. I know that living exemplary values is the road to fulfillment, and I know for certain we cannot take life or love for granted.

THERE'S NO DOUBT I feel great freedom as a self-proclaimed superhero—that many of the things that tend to weigh us down or trip us up as humans now seem trivial to me—but it does isolate me to a degree. Those of us lucky enough to survive nearly dying without long-lasting harm know what I mean. I don't judge people, but I do have trouble tolerating some of the petty concerns I hear.

"I need [this or that]. This one's already a year old."

"Did you see [insert name here] today? I cannot believe how he/she looks."

"I can't believe that play by [insert professional sports player name here]. What a joke!"

"I hate what [celebrity] named her/his baby. What were they thinking?"

The sheer number of inconsequential things people pay attention to, complain about, and take personally baffles me when what truly matters is the gift of life itself; the miracles of nature, the cosmos, and the human body; and striving to improve the quality of the lives of others by being compassionate, ferreting out injustice, and reducing suffering.

Many of my friends sense this change in me. Sadly, I have lost colleagues I mistook as friends, which I suspect is because they know I see through them. Or perhaps these friendships were always empty, but now with my clarity, I no longer see what I mistakenly thought was a constructive relationship. I take personal accountability for confusing fawning for friendship, but I'm also extremely grateful: I now have no problem discerning the people I can sincerely count on. Perhaps most interesting is that those friends with whom I now feel closer have themselves gone through significant personal trials. What we have in common is not only surviving the crucible but learning how to manage that new outcome for the better.

If you're finding yourself in a self-reflective space right now, contemplating your own values and what matters most to you, you may wish you had the Clarity of Vision superpower too. If so, I'm here to tell you that it's not exclusive to those who've survived a trauma—it's attainable by anyone who understands the concept of an inflection point, or the mathematical location whereby a curve suddenly changes its direction. In simple terms, it is my physical trauma that now serves as my personal inflection point—the point from which I changed my direction, or my thinking. But anyone can visualize a new directional outcome. It merely requires an infusion of energy toward your desired state of mind, dedication to maintaining it, and enjoying the outcome.

For me, it all comes back to the many times I had fantasized about trying to change the world, particularly the world of medicine. I have now been handed an opportunity—and even a platform—to attempt to instigate that change in a much more constructive manner than when I was taking it on by myself. That is the purpose of this book: to start multiple conversations on a national level about the current, often misguided, practice of conventional medicine, to upend inaccurate assumptions regarding its technology, and to expose surreptitious conflicts of interest.

Think how remarkable it would be if everyone could come together with their individual superpowers to make this sweeping, necessary, life-affirming change a reality.

◆

chapter twenty-one

ROSS

Jerusalem

At one point while I was in the rehabilitation facility, Denise and I agreed to take a vacation together, as we do most every year. But this time, it had deeper meaning: it would signify that I had survived the trauma and survived the treacherous journey back to a level of wellness that supported being able to travel.

After weighing numerous options, we decided on Israel. I jokingly labeled it my "Thank You Tour." What better way to recognize my amazing accomplishment than to visit this sacred land, I reasoned. Returning to normal was my primary goal, so to further inspire that achievement, we scheduled the trip for several months after my projected return home.

When the date of departure finally arrives, I am eager to put the reason for the trip behind me. I don't want to focus on the before, only the after. I hold strong to my new worldview— my Clarity of Vision—and set out to take in every detail of the Holy Land.

Though Denise and I come from different religions, we have great respect for both. When we make the trip to Galilee, I am moved at the sites where Jesus preached. When we travel to the Western Wall, Denise is moved by the significance of the

Jewish pilgrimage. But it is at the Wall that I personally have a spiritual experience.

Keeping with old religious tradition, the Wall is segregated: women are on one side and men on the other. On this particular morning, very few people dot the length of the historic site. I humbly walk toward an empty space, bow my head, and place both hands, fingers spread, flat upon the stones—the stones that remain of the retaining wall of the Temple Mount, which was destroyed by the Roman emperor's son, Titus, to quell the Jewish revolt in 70 CE.

With my eyes closed, I silence my brain. Suddenly, my mind is filled with the silent mantra I had played repeatedly in my head to get through the many painful procedures in the ICU and through my perpetual state of unrest in the hospital:

Help me, help me, help me, thank you, thank you, thank you.

I had forgotten about my desperate plea to a higher power for solace and peace during my hospitalization, and the acknowledgment that I could make it. This resurfacing moved me so deeply that tears welled and poured from my eyes. I was indeed lucky to have made it, and it was remarkable that the mantra had returned to me in this holy place.

But this wasn't the only poignant moment I experienced.

At the crypt of the Church of the Holy Sepulchre, pilgrims must typically wait in a seemingly unending line. To keep order when people finally reach the entrance, the priests who oversee the area usher people through, giving only a few seconds per person within the aedicule, or small shrine. The aedicule contains two rooms: the first holds the Angel's Stone, which is a fragment of a large stone that sealed Jesus's tomb; the second is the actual tomb of Jesus.

As Denise and I near the shrine, for some unknown reason, a Greek Orthodox priest holds the line by placing his hand before us. He then waves us through, but keeps those behind us back. We continue to snake our way to the entrance as two by two, people quickly enter and exit the aedicule, which holds six to eight people. By the time we enter the tomb of Jesus, we are stunned to discover that we're completely alone. Everyone else has exited, and no one new is entering. It is, without a doubt, the most surreal experience of my life, as if time has actually stood still. Denise is moved to tears as we take in the sacred moment that seems so divinely orchestrated just for us. No one rushes us, and no one joins us. We breathe in the pocket of time that will surely never be duplicated for the two of us alone. When we finally leave, time returns to normal and the priest lets the crowd surge forward again.

I have no rational explanation.

A similar experience occurs at the Tomb of the Virgin Mary. Despite the site's popularity, when we arrive, massive numbers of people are exiting the shrine. By the time we reach the bottom of the stairs and approach the inner chamber, we are again completely isolated, as if God has gently nudged everyone toward other sites to give this unrepeatable holy experience to Denise and me alone.

I have never been filled with more serenity, and I have never been more aware of pure, free-flowing grace.

My post-trauma self, having been given gifts beyond any expectation, undeniably sees the world through a very different pair of eyes.

ADVOCACY

The chapters that follow elucidate specific areas surrounding patient care in our country that would benefit from attention. My goal is to ignite awareness, which then sparks conversation, which then energizes the myriad of brilliant minds capable of reshaping the system, which then motivates the level of sweeping change so desperately required in our current medical establishment—one that will monumentally elevate the patient experience and healing journey, along with the physician's capacity to facilitate such an experience. This is demonstrated well in the Modern Hippocratic Oath that many doctors recite today in medical school, which was adapted from the original in the 1960s by academician, Dr. Louis Lasagna:

I swear to fulfill, to the best of my ability and judgment, this covenant:

I will respect the hard-won scientific gains of those physicians in whose steps I walk, and gladly share such knowledge as is mine with those who are to follow;

I will apply, for the benefit of the sick, all measures which are required, avoiding those twin traps of overtreatment and therapeutic nihilism.

I will remember that there is art to medicine as well as science, and that warmth, sympathy and understanding may outweigh the surgeon's knife or the chemist's drug.

I will not be ashamed to say "I know not," nor will I fail to call in my colleagues when the skills of another are needed for a patient's recovery.

I will respect the privacy of my patients, for their problems are not disclosed to me that the world may know. Most especially I must tread with care in matters of life and death. If it is given me to save a life, all thanks. But it may also be within my power to take a life; this awesome responsibility must be faced with great humbleness and awareness of my own frailty. Above all, I must not play at God.

I will remember that I do not treat a fever chart, a cancerous growth, but a sick human being, whose illness may affect the person's family and economic stability. My responsibility includes these related problems, if I am to care adequately for the sick.

I will prevent disease whenever I can, for prevention is preferable to cure.

I will remember that I remain a member of society, with special obligations to all my fellow human beings, those sound of mind and body, as well as the infirm.

If I do not violate this oath, may I enjoy life and art, respected while I live and remembered with affection hereafter. May I always act so as to preserve the finest traditions of my calling and may I long experience the joy of healing those who seek my help.

◆

chapter twenty-two

The Dangers of Labeling

You have heart disease.
You have irritable bowel syndrome.
You have stage IV cancer.
You have Alzheimer's.

What do you feel when you hear these diagnoses? I can almost guarantee it's a sense of dread. And why wouldn't it be? At this point in time, conventional medicine leans heavily on these labels, and there's rarely an encouraging statement that follows them.

While labeling a patient with an illness or disease is seemingly innocuous and necessary to determine a treatment protocol, it often causes unseen collateral damage to the patient. Whether the label is presented in layman's terms, such as my being told I had a traumatic brain injury (TBI), or it's delivered using some cumbersome moniker in Latin, such as dermatofibroma, what lurks under the label is almost always nebulous and scary to the patient. Something called a "traumatic brain injury" makes sense after a fall or blow to the head, but what does it *really* mean? Dermatofibroma is simply the Latin for "hard skin," but the Latin term sounds like an incurable disease of some kind.

The truth is, most illnesses have a root cause that doesn't

stem from an accident like mine. Symptoms are simply a manifestation of pathophysiology. This means that something is
wrong, usually on a cellular level. If we as physicians truly listen, we can often hear the body telling us exactly what that
something is. Physicians identify patterns—that's the crux of
our job. The problem is that once a pattern is identified and
subsequently labeled with a diagnosis, it does not necessarily
mean the patient will experience the anticipated outcome.

Over time, physicians have come up with all sorts of names
for illnesses we can't readily explain, and in doing so, we pass on
that label to the patient, who then takes on whatever fear and
negative aspects or outcomes are associated with that illness:
being put on medications with detrimental side effects, undergoing a toxic treatment plan with even scarier side effects, losing
physical or mental capacity, early or agonizing death, the list
goes on. Unfortunately, in the vast majority of cases, prescribing
pharmaceuticals or toxic protocols is the norm—and it's merely
an attempt to "offset" symptoms of that disease, which almost
always leaves the root cause unidentified, thereby prolonging the
patient's sickness. Sadly, this frequently results in even more
problems caused by what the prescribed chemicals do to their
system. This vicious cycle has led to patients having less and less
feeling of control over their own wellness because they're trusting those of us in white coats to know best.

In this twisted scheme of conventional-based care, I assert
that we can and do miss the mark.

As a result, patients suffer. And physicians, unwilling or
unable to address the true cause of the illness and therefore
execute the opposite of what the Modern Hippocratic Oath
pledges, suffer too.

❧

WE KNOW THAT the mind is extremely powerful. Giving someone a burdensome diagnosis—even if they don't have that disease—can actually cause symptoms to physically manifest, purely from the mind believing its presence to be true and harnessing fear of the symptoms, treatment, or outcome. This is not fluff; science has shown this and other outcomes of the placebo effect in numerous trials—both on the side of healing a disease, and on the side of triggering or exacerbating disease.

What the mind believes is real can become real.

Consider this:

I was told I had a traumatic brain injury (TBI), and just like that, I was labeled. The physicians on my team told me it would likely take a full year before the TBI settled down; my own parents took that as fact and believed I wouldn't be able to return to work as quickly as I planned. From then on, any decision I made that they felt they couldn't support became defined as a "result of my TBI." They even went so far as to ask my wife to hand over my legally owned guns. Because my brother read that people with TBI can become suicidal, he and my father singlehandedly decided it was appropriate to remove them from our home. While some people may interpret this as motivated by love and concern, I saw this as demonstrative of an inappropriate desire to control—fully supported by my new "label." They could have simply suggested to Denise that the guns be kept locked up for the time being, just in case. But to suggest that the guns be illegally forfeited to them was insulting. If I truly wished to kill myself, I could have effortlessly found other means of doing so. I share this to illustrate how well-intentioned family members can make matters worse by defining a patient only by his or her disease—or in my case, a result of my fall.

Physicians, steeped in their conditioned role, invariably do the same.

Now imagine a different scenario.

Instead of being told I had TBI, and saddling me with a potentially destructive label that carried numerous negative connotations, the doctors could easily have told me this:

> Ross, your head took a blow when you fell, and it's perfectly normal to be a bit out of sorts right now because of it. But your body is a remarkable self-healing vessel. We'll help you out with some cognitive therapy to get those synapses firing again the way they should. But there's no reason you shouldn't be back to your sharp, intelligent self in no time. Keep in mind, too, that our thoughts are immensely powerful. I recommend finding some affirmations that support your healing and saying them multiple times a day. Really take those words in as truth, and you'll help your healing process along tremendously.

If I asked how long they thought it would take, they could say:

> We hate to put a timeframe on healing, Ross, because each person is different. If we tell you it'll be a year and you believe that as fact, your mind might actually program itself to take that long. If we tell you two weeks and you're not quite back to speed that quickly, you may get down on yourself. So what we recommend is setting a goal in your mind that feels reasonable to you. Don't hold yourself back, and don't be too hard on yourself if you need a little more time. As I said, everyone is different. We'll be here to help you along with all aspects of your recuperation, but the best

thing to do is simply believe in yourself and your body's ability to heal. Both cognitive and physical therapies are excellent tools to help you, so use these techniques until you no longer need them. If you do that, there's really no limit on how quickly you can heal and get back to work.

Do you feel the difference between the two models of physician interaction?

One labels and *disempowers*; the other foregoes the label and *empowers*.

Lucky for me, I eschewed the labels and refused to be put into a box. I knew myself. I knew I could heal. I challenged my mind and body to achieve that. And I did it, in much less time than anyone predicted.

But most people, particularly when they're at their most vulnerable, don't have the strength, awareness, or wherewithal to shrug off a label and envision a different outcome from the one they've been told to expect.

This is one of the great tragedies of labeling a patient and that person internalizing it as fact (not to mention that people are often conditioned to receive "rewards" through labels, whether through sympathy or insurance payments).

A perfect example of an erroneous assumption based on a label was my being told that TBI would likely cause depression. There were numerous reasons I could have lapsed into depression: nearly dying and fearing for a time that there may not be a grander purpose to life; the feeling of abandonment when people I thought were true friends really weren't; realizing people's selfishness can be so pronounced that they cannot provide what's needed during someone's crisis. I also felt reduced to an unlucky metaphor when one of my physical therapists told me she yelled at her husband for wanting to work on their roof, referencing me as a cautionary tale. My Harvard and Yale educations, my professional accomplishments including publishing numerous manuscripts, my lifelong volunteer work overseas, seemed to become irrelevant overnight—I suddenly felt like the poster boy for carelessness or bad luck. But none of these feelings were caused by my brain being intensely scrambled. They were simply natural outcomes of surviving a traumatic event and having to take in people's response to it.

While there are certainly proven interventions required to take for specific illnesses that are life-saving, my point is that more often than not, we as physicians take the labeling route. We are also quick to prescribe the pharmaceutical—or worse, the "you have X amount of time"—route. This frequently harms patients rather than heals them. Let me repeat this: *This frequently harms patients rather than heals them.*

Once again, we as physicians must return to our Hippocratic Oath. When we do that and follow its precepts, we realize that any patient diagnosis calls for outlining *all* treatment options, with the risks and benefits of each. That may be challenging and time consuming to research and discern, but it's our responsibility to educate our patients and their families about the disease *and* its pathophysiology, not merely issue a label. In doing so, we allow enlightened patients to decide the course they wish to follow, help them understand the anticipated outcome, and work with them toward their wellness goal. When we *don't* do this—which is unfortunately the norm in modern medicine in this country—we leave our patients vulnerable, scared, and sometimes even bullied, instead of educated, encouraged, and empowered. Whether the drugs they're prescribed make them sicker in the long run, or they internalize the diagnosis as their doom, they are essentially stripped of potentially health-affirming options and the known healing benefit of optimism, both of which go a long way toward restoring a person's overall wellness.

I have spent a great deal of time trying to understand why many physicians do not behave this way—and one of the biggest reasons is how we are trained. Like an eager pre-med student taking the MCAT exam, we aggressively seek the right answer because that's how we win. But once we've completed our schooling, internship, and residency, we tend to continue seeking one-word answers as if taking a multiple-choice exam. We seek the response based only on a label or diagnosis: hypertension, endometriosis, melanoma, etc. Perhaps worse, *patients* have come to expect this as the norm. Once they receive the label, our information age has made it easy to research it on Google before they even reach their car in the parking lot, then internalize all the ways that exist to approach whatever "illness" they've been saddled with, particularly those that weren't discussed with their doctor. On one hand, this can be empowering; on the other, it can be terribly overwhelming.

Another problem is that physicians are not rewarded for exploring with patients how the labels they're given will forever change their lives—for the better or for the worse. Consider this: Most people don't think about it, but pregnancy is, in fact, a diagnosis. When women receive this news, however, they have multiple means of support to get them through the process, such as books, classes, online resources, family and friends who've had children, and so on. But when I deliver the label of dermatofibrosarcoma protuberans (which means hard skin and soft tissue sticking out of body cancer) to a patient, they don't have as many resources at their disposal to help them on their journey to wellness. I educate them about the relatively good prognosis and the surgery required to reach a

cure, and I spend time answering questions and being supportive, but the same infrastructure available to pregnant women
doesn't exist for these particular patients to address their
unique fears and concerns. This is why it's crucial that we as
doctors take the hands of our patients and talk to them about
all the options currently available to them, not simply the usual
pharmaceutical or surgical one.

As another example, I see many refractory wounds, or
rather wounds that don't respond to treatment, in patients
with diabetes. Whenever this occurs, I'm amazed at how little
understanding patients have about this disease—and I respond
by taking the time to give them critical information, relating to
them by sharing my personal experiences and that I, too, must
watch my processed sugar intake. This relatively minimal but
vital exchange has positively improved the lives of quite a few
of my patients with chronic wounds due to poorly controlled
diabetes. Simply spending time with them to explore the
meaning of their "label" and the action it takes to avoid problems, I find it's not uncommon, three months after an initial
meeting when a repeat HgA1c test is obtained (a test that reflects how well diabetes is controlled), that the patient has a
big smile and is proud of his or her improvement. Once again,
when patients become more empowered, they often begin to
take better care of themselves, which is a win-win for everyone.

Perhaps another contributing factor motivating physicians
to label patients is the protection from medicolegal ramifications that it grants. In other words, if a patient is given a poor
prognosis, the physician may feel he or she is protected to a
degree from a poor outcome and the family is therefore less
likely to sue. In my case, I imagine that my ICU team was
somewhat terrified that if they painted an optimistic picture,
and my outcome was much grimmer than they predicted,

Denise would have been angry. That wouldn't have been the case, but the common theory is that if the prognosis is dire and the outcome matches, or the outcome is better than the dire picture painted, no one can be upset. Unfortunately, this simply feeds the pessimistic paradigm that lends to deleterious labeling.

TO BRING THE message of this chapter to a close, I offer a brief story.

Plastic surgeons are required to pass a 200-question examination every ten years for re-certification. Just days before my trauma at the end of December, I signed up to take the exam in April, as my ten-year mark was approaching. While I was in the ICU, however, my team was so pessimistic about my prognosis that I started to doubt my own ability. In my physicians' opinions, I was cognitively unable to take that exam with TBI and likely would be for at least twelve months, so I asked Denise to contact the Board and put the exam on hold.

Had I listened to what the doctors told me, I might have believed I needed to wait an entire year. Instead, just a few months after my trauma, I confidently felt the neural network of my brain had returned to normal and scheduled the exam as initially planned when it was offered in April.

I earned a close to perfect score of 99 percent.

◆

chapter twenty-three

Rethinking Common Practices:
Endotracheal Intubation, Tracheostomy,
and Gastrostomy Tubes

During the time I was in the ICU, I had all three of the
title procedures: endotracheal intubation, tracheostomy,
and the placement of a gastrostomy tube. What you probably
don't know is how antiquated and problematic each of them is,
and how each one has affected me, probably for the rest of my
life.

ENDOTRACHEAL INTUBATION

While there's no doubt that intubation saves lives, the design
of the endotracheal tube dates from about the time we first
landed a man on the moon. With fifty years of technological
advances behind us, this begs the question: Why have we not
revisited this apparatus's fundamental design?

I know firsthand that being intubated is one of the worst,
most uncomfortable positions a conscious patient can be in. It
literally feels as if you're being choked at all times. It made me
so crazed that as you'll recall, I pulled the tube out myself as
soon as I was able. Once it was removed, I expected to feel
enormous relief, but the truth was that I had difficulty breath-

ing due to the multitude of rib fractures and needed the tube reinserted shortly thereafter.

Let me give you an illustration of what the endotracheal tube does to the throat.

Pressure sores have always been a problem for patients in prolonged hospital stays, or for those who aren't ambulatory. But we know these can be completely avoided by shifting the patient frequently and distributing weight off the skin in affected areas in defined intervals. I, for example, was shifted frequently during my three weeks in the ICU, and therefore did not develop any cutaneous pressure sores. My family understood the irony of a plastic surgeon suffering a pressure sore and frequently asked the nurses if I was being shifted accordingly. Fortunately, this particular ICU had a well-established protocol in place and followed it closely. For this, I was sincerely grateful.

But with intubation, patients are unable to tolerate shifting of the tube because it causes coughing. It may seem as though the tube is merely resting in the throat, but it's actually producing the same type of pressure on the mucosal lining that occurs on the skin when a patient is lying down. Therefore, there is a finite amount of time a patient can remain intubated before physicians worry about the patient developing a pressure sore within the throat. For this reason, we desperately need a new design, where pressure points can shift automatically over timed intervals along the length of the tube as it expands and collapses. I'm convinced that putting innovation into this would avoid a great deal of morbidity, and could potentially lend more long-term comfort and/or benefits to patients who are already in a profoundly uncomfortable state.

This leads me to tracheostomy.

TRACHEOSTOMY

Currently, forcing patients into tracheostomy after prolonged intubation is a classic nod to medical history—justified by the need to avoid the prolonged pressure that the endotracheal tube produces on the mucosa of the throat. If unrelieved, as I mentioned prior, this pressure causes necrosis. But, as I was to learn, a tracheostomy creates an entirely different set of problems.

Unfortunately, like with intubation, the tracheostomy procedure is outdated—the current technique was first described during the Roman Republic and refined during the Renaissance. What's more, although studies support early tracheostomy following endotracheal intubation for decreased risk of infection and narcotic usage, these studies are from the 1970s and '80s. The fact that we haven't revisited this procedure with modern methodology is tragic. A technique known as percutaneous dilatational tracheostomy is less invasive, yet although it is performed in some locations of the United States, it has not caught on. This begs investigation of why new technologies that are potentially significantly better are not adopted by surgeons in the US. This is precisely why I speculate that a mere redesign of the endotracheal tube could potentially avoid tracheostomy altogether, if the tube is designed in the way I described, or better.

As a trained otolaryngologist, I had always been told a tracheostomy is relatively well tolerated, yet nothing could be further from the truth. Although potentially lifesaving, the tracheostomy causes a persistent, painful issue while in place: the accumulation of a large amount of sputum. This may not seem like a painful problem until you understand that the suctioning necessary to remove it is nearly intolerable. Now imagine the angst a patient feels knowing this action is required every several hours.

In my case—which I know speaks for many others saddled with a trach—the kindest nurses and respiratory therapists used the red rubber catheter to gently clean around the tracheostomy, clearing the clogged mucous. The less kind ones rammed the catheter deep into my trachea and down my lungs, resulting in uncontrollable and spasmodic coughing that resembled grand mal seizures. A person would have to be superhuman to become accustomed to the deep pain this caused.

One respiratory therapist was particularly sadistic. Clearly a disgruntled human being with a chip on his shoulder, this man never explained what he was about to do and never apologized for the pain he caused. As he worked on me, he took personal calls on his cell phone. He smiled malevolently. His crowning achievement was that every time he walked past me, he would remove the cap from my tracheostomy and place it on the counter out of my reach. No words, no explanation. Just that damn smirk on his face. Of course, with the cap off, I was unable to speak. It wasn't until later I learned that weeks earlier, my father had complained to this therapist about his cleanliness while suctioning my tracheostomy. I guess this was his revenge.

I am sure there are rancorous people in every field. However, in medicine, we owe it to our patients to perform our best and to police those, like this man, who malign the system. I don't know if the hospital was short-staffed and relied on this person to fill in the gaps, but I do know he should have never been allowed to work with patients. Although his behavior was inappropriate, however, I felt too scared and vulnerable to complain. As horrible as it sounds, I could honestly imagine him suffocating me and claiming I aspirated, so I tolerated his torture quietly.

In the best-case scenario, a tracheostomy can eventually be removed when a person is safely off the ventilator. However, this process, known as decannulation, is not simple. For days afterward, as the hole slowly closes, it constantly leaks sputum. Once the hole finally seals, the larynx resides in a new position from the tethering of the scar. As a result, swallowing becomes an entirely new process; I've actually had to teach myself how to swallow certain foods differently. For example, when I eat ice cream now, the melting liquid hits my vocal cords and triggers spasmodic coughing, something I never experienced previously. Also, when I tilt my head downward, my voice becomes weaker, which affects how loudly I'm able to speak while performing surgeries. Again, this is because scar tissue now pulls at my larynx, which makes air escape past my vocal cords when I'm in this position, thus permanently changing the quality of my voice. Even with my head in a normal, upright position, my voice is often breathy and softer than before due to these scars.

Yes, it's despairing to have these repercussions of my trauma, but perhaps even more disconcerting is that as a trained otolaryngologist, I was never aware of the lifelong issues created by tracheostomy scars. Because of this, I simply followed the antiquated protocols and assumed patients would recover just fine.

I assumed the same about another under-studied practice: the placement of a gastrostomy tube.

GASTROSTOMY TUBE (PEG)

It is not uncommon for ICU patients to undergo both tracheostomy and percutaneous endoscopic gastrostomy tube (PEG) placement simultaneously, and I was no exception. Having these accoutrements typically facilitates transfer of the patient to a long-term care facility and out of the ICU. In the medical world, however, tracheostomy and PEG are typically reserved for "gomers" (Get Out of My Emergency Room, as per the famous book *House of God*) or "goners."

A PEG is a feeding tube that goes from the skin of the abdomen to the stomach, allowing liquid feedings that can't be taken by mouth, either due to sedation or a vegetative state. So when I overheard the physicians talking to Denise about this in my ICU bay, I felt immediately overtaken by desperation, thinking they saw me as someone who wouldn't recover. Deep inside, I had a gnawing fear that perhaps I overstayed my welcome in the ICU. I knew the pressure that physicians were under to move patients along to save the hospital money. Trach and PEG were procedures commonly performed to decrease the length of ICU stay. In fact, the medical acronym "TPK" was used in slang parlance for Trach PEG Kindred (a long-term acute-care facility). Remember, too, that although I was processing enough to hear and understand what was going on, I still felt completely disconnected from reality, as if everything was happening to someone else. I recall thinking there was no way I was actually going to undergo these procedures myself; I truly believed that I was trapped in an alternative universe, that it was all a dream I would wake up from at some point. In that state, I gave a literal thumbs up, as though acquiescing to merely another hurdle I needed to clear in order to get home. Since I wasn't in a state to question how many days had elapsed while I was intubated, or to distinguish reality from delusion, I projected the attitude of "Let's just knock it out." If I needed this procedure to expedite going home, I reasoned, I wanted to do it and move forward.

As predicted, the tracheostomy and PEG indeed expedited my release from the ICU, but I honestly question if these interventions were truly necessary to facilitate that release. Yes, I was decannulated shortly after the trach and PEG placement and was breathing on my own and eating (albeit small amounts). But, sadly, I feel the only reason I was decannulated was that I persistently questioned the need for these interventions—and more forcefully each day. Had I not been an advocate for myself with my knowledge as a physician, who knows how long I might have been kept on these protocols without merit. On the outside, I appeared to have a dire prognosis as a "severely impaired person with a brain injury." Yet, as I've stated repeatedly, that label didn't reflect the entire picture of me at all. I was most definitely *not* a goner; I believe the trach and PEG were insisted upon by rote, not by logic.

Not only were these apparatuses left in place due to old-school thinking, but also as yet another reflection of the medicolegal monster rearing its ugly head. I had no indication that the team was motivated to remove these devices, likely because they were afraid of a negative outcome that would put them at fault. I was even discharged from inpatient rehabilitation with the feeding tube, though I had not used it since my arrival—and even though my physicians there were willing to pull the PEG out before I left. Why didn't they? Because the GI doctor firmly demanded that *he* would do it, despite the fact that I hadn't seen him since my departure from the ICU. Furthermore, because of poor communication and absence of any universal documentation, when I saw another well-qualified GI doctor as an outpatient, he was equally reluctant (appropriately) to pull the tube, saying he was unsure which type of tube was used. I can only imagine how long this process would have taken had I not been a physician myself.

Even when I was at in-patient rehab, the number of people with capped trachs who never used them was remarkable. And I certainly cannot venture a guess of how many of my rehab classmates had unused PEGs hidden underneath their shirts and gowns. These accoutrements simply kept people defined as a patient and prevented them from any semblance of feeling normal, while permitting physicians to feel legally protected in the unlikely event these devices were needed.

And the problems the PEG created cannot be overlooked either. This is a further example of a procedure that is not as benign as physicians think. Case in point: Even though the PEG is now removed, there is a significant scar along my abdominal musculature where the tube exited. When I perform a crunch there is a palpable knot, which is presumably scar tissue in the muscle where the tube penetrated. Although this lump itself is of no consequence, the patch of scar in the muscle *is* an issue. This is because when I lift something heavy, the scar triggers significant fibrillations of the muscle and results in significant pain. Even stifling a sneeze can trigger these painful muscle spasms. As a result, just as I had to learn how to swallow certain foods to avoid coughing spells, I had to do the same with heavy lifting and sneezing.

As I indicated before, despite having a PEG, I still lost a significant amount of muscle mass from prolonged immobility. Two factors permitted the loss of muscle in my case as an immobilized patient in the ICU: 1) lack of adequate nutritional intake; and 2) absence of muscle exercise. Although I was seen by nutritionists and feeding formulas were calculated, it was clearly not enough. To prevent muscle loss, patients require adequate nutrition to counteract the significant catabolic (metabolic breakdown) stressors of illness. If the team does not have top-notch nutritionists accurately calculating these complex requirements daily and guaranteeing patients receive the needed supplementation through various means, massive wasting will occur.

In short, since an immobilized patient cannot actively exercise muscles, the other important aspect of preventing muscle wasting is eliminated.

But what about electrical stimulation? There are indeed multiple studies in the scientific literature demonstrating how neuromuscular electrical stimulation of immobilized patients stimulates muscle building and prevents disuse atrophy. However, this has not yet caught on in the ICUs of our country. Think about that. We have both the studies and technology to prevent muscle atrophy in those individuals who are wasting away in the ICU but do not make it a reality. I have no idea why, but I could venture a guess: costs. (Ironically, neuromuscular electrical stimulation is used in some medical spas to passively create a "six-pack" abdomen for paying clients, yet we do not have this in ICUs for deteriorating patients.)

The bottom line is: a yet-to-be-invented modern design of the endotracheal tube could have allowed me to avoid tracheostomy or PEG for a few days longer, or possibly altogether, enabling me to escape significant cicatricial—or scar-related—consequences during my recovery. Furthermore, an already existing and proven technology of neuromuscular electrical stimulation combined with aggressive nutritional support could have saved me from losing a significant amount of muscle strength, which required weeks to rebuild.

Tracheostomy and PEG are clearly needed for some patients, but I believe we must be much more prudent about when and why we make those decisions for individual patients, and much more passionate about modernizing each of these interventions. Further, muscle wasting in immobilized patients could be dramatically lessened by strictly applying the outcome of complex mathematical calculations while simultaneously utilizing medical devices that already exist. We simply have to make it a priority of healthcare.

chapter twenty-four

Re-Examining the ICU

Coming in and out of heavy sedation. Round-the-clock sounds emitting from multiple machines. Frequent waking by nurses. An excess of uncomfortable wires and tubes. Persistent nightmares.

This is the current ICU environment in the majority of hospitals in our country.

While it's sad to say—and while life-saving measures certainly do occur—if you've never required care in an ICU, count yourself highly fortunate and be grateful. Although patients do recover, and I was one of those people, I can, without reservation, say that virtually nothing about the ICU environment supports healing. I realize it may sound extreme, but I am not exaggerating when I compare the ICU to prison. I am certain that ICU patients experience torture similar to inmates in solitary confinement, where the forced isolation does nothing to improve the person's mind, body, or spirit; in fact, it serves to do the opposite. The ICU is structured in much the same way. This chapter is therefore my critical call to the medical community for a massive overhaul of the ICU, with the goal of providing an environment exponentially more conducive to calm, stress-free, restful healing while receiving necessary medical attention.

SUPPORTING A HEALING EXPERIENCE

Imagine being admitted to a hospital with serene, homelike surroundings. You have a private room with an extra bed for your spouse, partner, or loved one to stay with you at all times. If you need to be connected to a machine or two, they're powered by wireless technology and only make a sound if an emergency arises. Restraints of any kind are not allowed. Sedation is used only when necessary for pain and in responsible moderation, and an uninterrupted, good night's rest is not only encouraged but supported by privacy and quiet. The vibrant facility is fully staffed around the clock with physicians, nurses, and therapists trained in the compassionate arts, as well as in the medical arts; everyone addresses you by name, whether you're able to respond or not, and no procedure takes place without the utmost respect for your dignity and humanity. The staff is there to support your healing journey, and everything from the encouragement with which they speak to the kind way they handle delicate tasks to the attention they pay to what best serves you day to day toward your recovery is executed with optimism. And they don't simply address symptoms with surgery or pharmaceuticals; they seek to address the cause, while also ameliorating your spiritual and emotional health, as both play a vital role in your healing journey.

If this sounds excessively ideal, I can assure you it's not.

In fact, patient-centered facilities with many of these characteristics exist throughout the world, where thousands of patients each year flock for holistic treatment of cancer and other diseases. Why are these facilities almost exclusively overseas? Because sadly, they don't fit into the Big Pharma–controlled landscape in America.

I will concede that ICU patients and holistic cancer clinic patients may vary in the level of critical care needs, but the premise of the environment described nonetheless applies to both: patients need a truly healing *environment* if our jobs are to help them heal.

In my case, as you've read throughout this book, I was frustrated by countless elements that made my time in the ICU a living hell. But one of the worst was that my wife was not allowed to stay in my room overnight, which would have given me a great deal of comfort while significantly decreasing her stress. Visiting hours are in place to benefit the staff, not the patients; when a patient is ill enough to require life-saving measures, he or she needs a constant loving presence more than ever. I understand that the medical team must sometimes perform interventions that a family should not witness, but to forbid them from supporting their loved one 24/7 is illogical; family members can be politely escorted away when emergent procedures are performed.

It's further ridiculous to believe that patients won't receive needed rest at night if family are at the bedside. I was given massive doses of narcotics to stay quiet overnight; how much better would it have been for my wife to be there to reorient me when I awoke in confusion, rather than the night nurse simply telling Denise when she arrived in the morning that I was agitated? My wife's hand on my forehead would have been much more positive than a nurse pushing more fentanyl.

Beyond the physical, ICU patients and their families need emotional and spiritual support, but this is simply not our standard of care, and these topics were never addressed by my medical team. (Chapter Twenty-Five offers an extended discussion of this topic.) I have no doubt, and I'm sure hundreds of thousands of patients and their families would agree, that having trained counselors lead support groups for families of ICU patients would be immensely beneficial. These sessions could be offered during the nurses' shift change, when families are asked to leave the ICU, and not only address emotional issues, but also provide information about managing insurance or disability claims, all of which can be a heavy burden.

And let's not overlook the ratio of nurses to patients in the ICU. Although it's higher than in the general ward, it is not 1:1. This means that one nurse is likely overseeing two patients in the ICU simultaneously. While this may be manageable, God forbid both patients crash and a nurse is faced with Sophie's choice: which patient do I save? And when two gravely ill individuals are being nursed by one person, communicable diseases can accidentally spread, not to mention medication dosage errors and patient falls. This is precisely how I fell—my nurse was tending to her other patient.

If it's money that prevents 1:1 care in the ICU across America, as well as transforming it into an environment much more conducive to healing, it goes without saying that we need to refocus our goals.

THE DELETERIOUS EFFECTS OF OVER-SEDATION

While I was in the ICU, I experienced a phenomenon known as ICU delirium. Simply stated, your brain is unable to anchor to anything familiar. In my particular situation, when I was finally alert enough to interact sensibly, I had little idea where I was. My brain had caught snippets of my actual situation and subsequently created a delusional scenario, striving to make sense of the random data that penetrated my drug-induced fog. In other words, it was trying to process the passage of time and all the events I experienced while drifting in and out of awareness.

For example, you may recall three of several delusional dreams I described in Chapter Five.

In one, I was severely constipated and believed I had to use my fingers to dislodge an enormous bowel movement. When I reached in and pulled it out, it was attached to a string that seemed to never end. When I was later told by Denise that I had a rectal tube, this psychosis made much more sense.

In another, I was trapped in the seatbelt of the driver's seat, dangling upside down after an accident. When my car flipped, a football flew from the dashboard and lodged in my throat. I opened my mouth, grabbed the football, and pulled it out. I believed I had to do it to stay alive. Again, after a later discussion with Denise, I realized this was when I self-extubated my endotracheal tube.

In yet another disturbing dream, I truly believed I had to perform a challenging major surgical procedure in under an hour, and that although I was working as fast as I could, something wasn't working and I had to start over. In the *Matrix*-like reality of the narcotic fog I was under, my brain was working overtime to make sense of the sensory snippets I was receiving. This dream could have occurred during my rib plating procedure, as it was complicated by several pneumothoraxes that required further work. Or, more likely, it occurred during one of the multiple times I required an urgent intubation for respiratory failure.

All of this inability to anchor to reality as a result of what I believe was excessive sedation robbed me of time I could have spent using my mind to help myself heal.

Sedation is also a significant problem when patients are hooked to a ventilator. Because the discomfort is nearly unbearable, sedation is frequently required if a patient is lucid, as almost everyone will fight the smothering presence of the tube. But instead of merely calming a patient, nurses will sometimes heavily sedate him or her so there is no resistance whatsoever. Although the amount of sedation used for a given patient should arguably be similar at all hours of the day, healthcare workers will often state that the patient was agitated and required more sedation at night. I question the veracity of this, as I've experienced firsthand that night staff might simply want a relaxed shift without issues. The heavy sedation, along with restraints, ensures no patient will have the opportunity to "get agitated." This is yet another reason we must insist on proper advocacy when it comes to sedation. Our objective must always be preserving a patient's humanity, not merely viewing them as a body we can do with what we wish, simply because it's more convenient. As such, I propose that an advocate should monitor and review daily how much sedation has been used for all ICU patients. Sudden bumps in use may point to a team member over-utilizing these drugs for a patient.

And let's be clear about the subject of sleep. A wide swath of our population touts the little amount of sleep they get as somehow admirable. This has diminished the crucial role sleep plays in our optimal level of health. Our own medical students are pushed to the brink with authority-imposed sleep deprivation. But I can tell you that operating on very little sleep is not a badge of honor, or in any way admirable; it's actually quite the opposite.

We know for a fact that rejuvenation of the body's cells and organs happens during sleep—not the kind of drug-induced sleep so prevalent in the ICU, but true, uninterrupted REM sleep—and that a persistent, or even temporary, lack of good sleep is harmful to the mind and body. How can anyone hope to heal, then, when night after night, for days or weeks on end, they're sedated into a sleep that doesn't serve the body's healing mechanisms?

The short answer is: they can't.

In my case, I attribute my quick recovery to my wife's demanding that the physicians stop administering so many narcotics and sleep aids to me. For this, and so many other things Denise demanded on my behalf, I am forever grateful to her.

RETURNING TO THE comparison I made earlier between the ICU and more patient-centered facilities, imagine if our own country's ICUs, and indeed our hospitals overall, operated in this fashion: patient—not profit—centered. Having been in an American ICU for three weeks, I can honestly say it can't happen soon enough.

◆

chapter twenty-five

The Importance of
Emotional Support

I touched on this topic in the previous chapter, but it's so critical that it merits its own chapter broken down into specific categories.

EMOTIONAL SUPPORT FROM HOSPITAL STAFF

While we are only now coming to appreciate the connection between emotions and recovery, there is no doubt that emotional support plays a profound role. Had Denise not been present at the hospital day in and day out to offer this support to me, I would have received little to none in the ICU.

Many of those who enter the medical field truly wish to ease suffering. The healthcare worker, though, must remember that he or she is fortunate enough to go home and relax with a spouse after pulling a grueling shift. He or she may even get a break for 15 minutes sometime during the day. As a patient, however, this is a 24/7 experience. I don't mean to minimize the remarkable human beings who work in the medical field and show sincere compassion for patients, but I must be honest and say that during my stay in the hospital, this was not always the case. Sometimes, I felt like I was merely on the receiving end of a job the person was required to do. *Check a vital. Push a button on a machine. Adjust a tube. Shift my position.* There were occasions where the person didn't even speak to me. It was as if to some, I quickly became just a body that no one saw as a person anymore. I am sure a factor is that some of these medical personnel feel drained being part of a broken system, but they must never forget that a fellow human being is on the receiving end of these actions.

We must also be real about the fact that a patient's immediate objective may be different from that of the medical team. Of course they wanted me healthy too, but members of the team each have competing personal goals that vie for their attention—ones that often differ significantly from the patient's. To give you a sense of what those goals might be, here's a short list:

Impress the chief medical officer
Make enough money by earning more Relative Value Units (RVUs), used in the United States Medicare reimbursement formula
Get home to my spouse tonight in time for dinner
Get through patient rounds and eat breakfast
Finish updating my medical records
Move on to the next patient who is sicker
Distribute all these medications accurately in the time allotted
Make the chief of service happy

While mine and other patients' healing journeys should be the top priority, these are actual thoughts in team members' heads against which patients must compete. I felt we were in daily hand-to-hand combat to redirect the staff's focus onto me so I could get out of the ICU in the best condition possible.

While I certainly appreciated the individuals who regularly brought compassion to the ICU each day, one thing is abundantly clear: we must create mandatory training for all healthcare workers on how to communicate more compassionately with severely ill patients, or with any patient for that matter. The particular skills of what these people do are indeed important, but their ability to connect on a human level is equally important. For example, just before a finger stick, or tracheal suction, various healthcare workers would say "I'm sorry" to me. Sometimes they said it with feeling; other times it was rote. In either case, they didn't use my name, and the words didn't convey what was going to happen or a sincere feeling of "sorrow" for the pain they were about to cause me. What would have given me much more solace was an honest and compassion conversation like this:

> "I'm so sorry about this, Ross . . . but I need to get some fresh oxygenated blood from the radial artery in your wrist. I know the needle looks scary, and I wish it weren't going to be painful, but the truth is that even though I'll be as gentle as possible, you're going to feel some discomfort. It should only last about [X] seconds, so if you can just breathe through it with deep five-second inhales and then five-second exhales through the nose when I give you the cue, that should help get you through it. And I'm sorry to add one more rough bit to this, but I should be honest and tell you this particular procedure may leave a permanent scar. It should be small, and the pain certainly won't last, but I just wanted you to have an honest picture of the whole procedure first."

The healthcare worker could then do one or two rounds of five-second deep breaths with the patient (provided the patient isn't on a ventilator; there would be an alternative calming method in that case), perhaps holding the person's hand for comfort. Once the patient felt a bit more at ease, the procedure could then begin.

Can you internalize the difference between this type of exchange before a procedure—particularly a painful one—versus a perfunctory "I'm sorry" on the part of the healthcare worker? Transparency, delivered with compassion and physical touch, could make all the difference in the patient's experience. I see no reason whatsoever why targeted training in how to speak with care and concern for patients, both when performing different procedures and when simply interacting, cannot be the standard for all types of medical programs—and thus become our normal and expected manner for engaging with patients.

Once again, a patient is a human being, regardless of how lucid, ill, or able to communicate (or not) they may be, and we must recognize the need for medical personnel to be trained in what we should call the "compassionate arts" to acknowledge this before all else.

EMOTIONAL SUPPORT FROM FAMILY

Unfortunately, in my case, it wasn't only certain staff who failed to see the importance of offering emotional support to me. Instead of holding my hand or stroking my head, my mother would merely wave from the foot of the bed and say hello. "I don't want to touch you in case I have a cold or the flu," she'd say. My father's way of coping was to bury himself in his work, which absolved him of having to make prolonged visits. While I imagined these were defensive moves on their part to protect themselves from the grief of my trauma, they had no idea how hurtful their distance was. During that time, more than any other in my life, I needed my parents to overlook whatever discomfort they might have felt in favor of providing me with the emotional support I desperately needed. Even a light touch and some verbal encouragement would have gone a long way.

In contrast, Denise's presence was like an arm reaching through a cloudy sky and pulling me to safety. I've elaborated throughout this book about the unceasing comfort and support my wife gave to me on a daily basis, but I truly can't emphasize enough what it meant to me and what a difference it made. She took so much ownership of my care that during a follow-up examination six months after my fall, she referenced when "we got home from rehabilitation." *We.* This is precisely why I recovered so well and so quickly: my partner was my advocate to such an extreme that she, too, felt like she had gone through my rehabilitation. To this day, I think of how faithfully she stood by me and the bliss it gave me.

SPIRITUAL SUPPORT

It speaks volumes that aside from my treasured time with Denise each day, visits with the chaplains were those I most looked forward to. This is ironic, as I am not particularly religious, but it goes to show how profoundly I craved the feeling that someone was rooting for me—particularly someone I didn't even know. This brought me so much strength that I played the odds: I am Jewish by birth, but I invited both Protestant ministers and Catholic priests to pray when they visited; I would have accepted the well wishes of an imam if one had come. My brother, perhaps upset that our religion was not represented, had his rabbi come. I view God as fickle, but I clearly needed his or her support in my time of need. *Now is no time to piss him or her off*, I reasoned tongue in cheek.

The truth is, adding prayer to a patient's daily medication list can't hurt. In fact, I believe it does more good than any of us knows. Anything that reinforces a person's faith, whether in the Divine or in their own ability to heal, has merit. We live in a politically correct climate today where not all patients may be comfortable with "God-talk," but many people derive strength precisely from their connection with a force greater than themselves. This may be rooted in a particular religion, or it may not. Either way, I propose that a spiritually based visit to each patient's room daily would serve to provide additional "medicine" that has been overlooked for far too long.

PROFESSIONAL EMOTIONAL SUPPORT

In Chapter Seventeen, I described the effects I experienced of PICS[1], or post-intensive care syndrome, which manifests in triggers and irrational fears from being in the ICU, such as sensitivity to certain sounds, a fear of isolation, or physical reminders of the ICU stay, like certain scars or marks.

In my review of the literature, physicians familiar with PICS recommend identifying those at risk and plugging them early into an environment of emotional support. They further encourage follow-up with survivors after discharge. The reality, however, is that these types of interventions may exist in acad-

---

[1] Having been through PICS myself, I now believe post-intensive care syndrome is an inaccurate description; it should reflect both the period in the ICU as well as after, which is why I suggest changing the term to "peri- and post-intensive care syndrome," or PPICS.

emic centers, but they don't exist in the real world. Whether it's because financial costs become prohibitive in a suburban or rural setting, or it is simply not a priority, enough attention is not paid to patients or to the family members who have survived the trauma with them. Denise and I could certainly have benefited from at least a few meetings to vent our frustrations and receive guidance from those who preceded us on this particular journey, but that support was not available.

The closest we got was in the rehabilitation facility, where they had a resident psychotherapist. This nod toward the difficulty of recovery was indeed helpful, but it was only a perfunctory nod; both Denise and I would have appreciated having a lot more time with her than we did. What little time I did spend with her was helpful, but perhaps Denise was helped even more. Although my fall was in no way her fault, Denise blamed herself to a degree, since she was the one who had pointed out the leak from the skylight. And my life wasn't the only one drastically altered, even if only for a relatively brief time, Denise's was too. (Ironically, the therapist was out of network and we received a large bill as a result.)

I would add that professional support would also be extremely helpful for those who require assistance with things like insurance, finances, or other private matters. These issues are immensely draining emotionally, particularly when health and medical issues are pressing as well. As such, I suggest we enact some type of program that engages experts in these fields who are willing to give time to helping patients who don't have family or other support—or who do have a loved one, as I did, but that person could use help in navigating the seemingly unending piles of paperwork involved in supporting a patient. What an incredible difference it would make to patients— young, old, or in between, isolated or not—to have someone there to support them through this overwhelming time, when so many critical decisions hang in the balance.

For all these reasons, we simply must amplify our focus on ensuring both patients and family members receive the emotional support from professionals they need.

EMOTIONAL SUPPORT FROM CARING INDIVIDUALS

I was fortunate to have my wife by my side as my champion, but not all ICU patients have family to advocate for them, and so they're simply left to blindly trust the system.

Feeling alone and abandoned is the hardest part of being a patient in the ICU. When visiting hours were over and Denise was required to leave, there were times that I cried. Being alone can lead to thoughts such as, *What is the point of going on?* And I *had* an amazing support system in Denise. Imagine having no one by your side to ease your fears or thoughts of resignation. Even worse, when we consider that many ICU patients are elderly and weak, the situation becomes even graver. Medical teams are sometimes dismissive of these people, believing that death is inevitable for elderly patients.

Every patient needs someone to watch over them, but these patients in particular are in need of an angel in the form of a human. For me, Denise served that role. She was there from before visiting hours started until she was forced to leave after they ended. She also took family leave, which was a difficult decision, as she is as much of a workaholic as I am. But she knew no one else would possibly look out for me like she would. She made the hospital staff feel as if they were directly accountable to her, and as a result, I received better and more meticulous care than I would have otherwise. I am certain this helped my recovery tremendously, which is why I propose at the very least, encouraging a new hospital volunteer program that mirrors one already in existence: Baby Cuddlers.

Baby Cuddlers—also called Rockers or Huggers—are hospital volunteers extensively trained in Neonatal Intensive Care Units across the country. All hospitals require these specialized volunteers to attend specific training, which prepares them to provide therapeutic talk and touch so necessary to early development. By simply holding the infants and reading, talking, or singing to them when the families can't be at the hospital because of work, school, or other childcare commitments, they play a crucial role in providing much-needed physical contact.

In the same way, I propose that volunteers could be trained as ICU Hand-Holders, people who spend loving, quality time with ICU patients who don't have constant support from a loved one. Imagine what a difference it could make to an elderly person in the ICU, or to a patient who doesn't have a support system nearby, to have someone hold their hand, to hear a soothing voice speaking encouraging words or reading to them, or to simply have a caring human by their side to let them know they're not alone.

Although audio therapy is a known technique in the ICU, it is not universally accepted in the conventional medical world. But through this proposed volunteer program, and through teaching physicians the importance of making sure only positive stimuli reach patients, I am convinced we could transform the ICU experience from a nightmarish one to a life-affirming and healing one. Although I cannot prove my wife's positive energy helped me, I know it was there because I could feel it. All ICU patients, who are undoubtedly in one of the most vulnerable and frightening situations of their lives, deserve the same positivity around them.

And this can be extended to all hospital patients—through volunteers who, instead of merely wheeling patients around, can be at the side of patients, offering uplifting conversation and emotional support. Anyone from high school students to older adults could be easily screened, and if approved, receive a one-day training with role-modeling activities to demonstrate appropriate ways to support patients emotionally. Millions of people in this country would love to feel they're making a difference through volunteering, and many of them would be perfectly suited to an opportunity such as this.

HOPE AND COMPASSION OVER FEAR OF LITIGATION

What all people need most when they're trying to survive a medical emergency is hope. Of course there is a time for somber honesty, but that doesn't mean physicians shouldn't speak words that inspire, not depress, at times of tragedy. We must never lose sight that miracles indeed occur daily. Sadly, this exchange of optimism is rarely what transpires in a medical setting.

For one, compassion isn't taught in medical school, and for some people, it *can't* be taught; some people's personalities are simply more scientific than they are caring. But if a doctor, nurse, or other technician is going to work directly with patients and not in a lab, learning how to talk to patients with positivity and compassion is a non-negotiable necessity: it simply must be as vital a part of one's medical training as the technical.

Second, with the fear injected into all medical personnel with regard to malpractice suits, I believe that fear of litigation—that if things turn out differently than a physician proposes—prevents doctors and nurses from projecting words of optimism that patients and families desperately need to hear. Robbing these people of hope may be an excellent legal defense, but it is by no means a practice of proper medicine. How many patients have given up hope because of defensive medical personnel? How many people could be happily reunited with family but instead fester in facilities because physicians fail to administer hope as medicine from fear of litigation?

FINALLY, I'VE SAID it before: Why hospitals behave like jails is beyond my comprehension.

There is not a single individual who spends time as an ICU patient who doesn't crave, and wouldn't benefit from, emotional support. This support should flow from hospital staff, family, professionals, spiritual leaders, and caring volunteers. The same is true for those who love them and sit vigil at the bedside.

It's time to make this the standard in our country, not the exception.

◆

chapter twenty-six

Preserving Dignity and Humanity

I f you recall my brief but raw illustration of the "pleasures" of ICU hygiene in Chapter Eleven, you know that anyone who has spent a stint in the hospital, particularly in the ICU, will tell you that modesty is difficult to cling to. While this may seem secondary in the face of potentially life-saving measures, it is nonetheless one of the numerous situations that puts patients in the most vulnerable of positions physically, where a healthcare worker becomes privy to bodily functions that would typically remain private: using a urinal or bedpan, having an enema or rectal tube, being changed into or out of a gown, wearing adult diapers or pads, being bathed, and urine or fecal accidents.

None of these scenarios are pleasant for either party, but they are particularly unpleasant for the majority of patients. Yet how diligently do most doctors, nurses, and technicians strive to preserve their patients' dignity? Certainly some do, but from my experience, those people were the exception, not the rule. This is why I assert that it is incumbent upon us in the medical profession to make preserving dignity a standard, as much as humanly possible. And because these situations arise daily, I believe it's important to explain precisely what preserving one's dignity must encompass.

PRIVACY

While more intimate contact with patients, such as the situations listed above, is typically performed behind a closed curtain, the truth is that curtain may only provide a thin veil of privacy, particularly if others share the room, or if other hospital staff are present. We should therefore be cognizant of the loudness with which we speak to a patient during a sensitive procedure. Having a nurse say "Oh, you made quite a mess" for everyone to hear, or "It's time for your enema!" is no one's business but the patient's. Simply using a softer voice, provided the patient can hear, lets a patient know we understand the awkwardness they're feeling, and it keeps the conversation contained between us and the patient as much as possible. In other words, not everyone in the vicinity hears that the patient is using the bedpan, having a diaper change, or experiencing any number of other private endeavors.

This is true when communicating with the patient's family members too. Whenever I speak to family who are sitting in a crowded waiting room before or after performing surgery, I ask them to step away so we can talk privately. Oftentimes they take this as a sign they're about to hear something tragic—which is sometimes the case—but more often than not, I'm able to reassure them I simply want to respect their privacy and that of their loved one. Unfortunately, many hospitals don't have a private area for family near the waiting room, and even when they do, surgeons are typically so rushed they don't take the needed time to shepherd a family into a truly private setting. From the feedback I've received from patients over and over again, however, the short amount of time it takes for a physician to usher loved ones to a quiet spot, and the gesture of sensitivity it carries, makes a world of difference to family and friends who are at once concerned and hopeful about the news they're about to receive.

RESPECTING MODESTY

You may recall something one of my patients said to me shortly after my return to work:

"As the doc knows, modesty is no longer an issue after what we've been through."

In a hospital environment, personal modesty is indeed something that often goes by the wayside; numerous patients are diminished to being essentially treated like an infant. Yet no health professional should take lightly how humiliating that is for an adult.

While revealing nakedness is unavoidable when patients are physically compromised, we can still approach the situation with respect and empathy, knowing that most people are uncomfortable being seen unclothed. Whether it's during a sponge bath, a bowel movement, an examination, or changing a gown, we should aim to respectfully keep patients appropriately covered with a towel, sheet, or blanket, or at least protect their modesty to the best of our ability. That simple, yet powerful gesture shows that we honor their sense of dignity, which heightens the level of caring our patients deserve, rather than merely seeing them as a body receiving perfunctory services. In the best cases, a particular nurse or technician may perform the same tasks for a patient on a regular basis, and a trust and comfort may form between this person and the patient. But because this is not always the case—and even when it is, the particular task may still be no less humiliating for the patient—it's at least helpful to have a caring individual who understands how delicate a position the patient is in.

I am so passionate about this that when I mark a patient before surgery in the holding area, if there is a risk of embarrassing bodily exposure, I insist the nurses place a sign on the curtain stating "procedure in process." This was something I did before my own personal experiences validated the importance of it. Many times, I had an impatient healthcare worker rip back a curtain, exposing a breast to the entire room while I marked it for a procedure. This is simply not appropriate.

Which leads me to preserving dignity's partner: humanity.

PRESERVING HUMANITY

I was recently in a skilled nursing facility early in the morning to remove a patient's sutures from a surgery I'd performed for a deeply invasive skin cancer. When I arrived, I immediately noticed that in every room, the beds were lowered nearly to ground level.

"Why are the beds so low?" I asked the nurse who was escorting me.

She explained that the state of New Jersey had forbid the use of side rails on beds because they are considered a form of restraint. I felt a smirk crawl across my face as post-traumatic stress disorder leapt up like a demon: I was instantly catapulted to being confined to my bed by disgruntled staff many nights during my rehabilitation experience. *Why was this allowed*, I wondered, *if state law forbids it?* In this facility, it was clear they had abided by the law *and* devised a reasonable solution to reducing the threat of patient falls; beds are designed with a mechanism that allows them to be lowered at night, so that if a patient did fall out of bed, it would be no more than four or six inches to the floor. In the morning, the bed can be easily raised to a normal height within minutes for the duration of the day.

As I watched her demonstrate this with my patient, I couldn't help but remember that not only was I tied down and sedated in the ICU, but I was also confined by bedrails during inpatient rehab. And make no mistake: these restraints are cruel. Secured with Velcro at the wrist and a snare wrap at the bedside, they are cinched so tightly that the patient cannot raise his or her hands, let alone scratch an itch or simply roll over in bed. I can attest to the fact that this is not only demeaning but also torturous. When I was lucid enough to understand I'd been restrained in this manner, I spent hours trying to escape. Denise even caught me one day hunched over the restraints trying to use my teeth to loosen the Velcro at my wrist like a wild dog. How we can justify treating patients this way is beyond my comprehension.

Managing overactive patients by sedating them with drugs and/or tying them up like an animal completely strips a patient of his or her humanity. I challenge anyone in the medical profession to be put in this position for a single day and not come out with the same stark realization that we simply cannot go on handling patients in this manner. In fact, I suggest that every medical student spend a few hours as a restrained patient—in a realistic ICU setting—to understand what it's like in our current system before they're able to graduate. We practiced blood draws and even prostate examinations on each other in medical school (I elected not to volunteer for the latter), so why not this? I believe this meaningful exercise would be but one step toward physicians leading the charge for more humane methods.

The excess use of sedation is another pressing problem. While this may be necessary when patients are in horrible pain, overly sedating them with drugs clouds their brains and, in my opinion, prolongs any hope of recovery. Furthermore, with the opioid crisis, we must take seriously the eschewing of unneces-

sary narcotics. In my case, despite the fog, I repeatedly asked
Denise and wrote dozens of times in my many notes to her to
help me feel "less drunk." She therefore demanded the minimal
amount of sedation possible to help move my recovery along; for
the medical staff, that meant physically immobilizing me with
medical restraints to keep me from trying to "go rogue." This
brings me back to the proposal I made in Chapter Twenty-Five
of creating a program to train volunteers as "ICU Hand-
Holders." These people could both comfort and watch over patients; if there was a problem with agitation or pain, the volunteer could summon a nurse. Not only would this minimize—or
better, eliminate—the need for any kind of physical restraints,
the patient would have a kind soul to offer them companionship
and comfort in their time of greatest need. As night shifts may
be more challenging to fill with volunteers, those shifts could
potentially be paid for by the hospital—provided these paid volunteers complete the same training as the unpaid volunteers,
and ensuring there are parameters in place for careful screening
to avoid potentially hiring people solely looking to make money.
I had Denise by my side thirteen hours a day, nearly every day,
but in the absence of my wife (which again, should not be the
hospital's decision; a spouse, partner, or other loved one should
be allowed to be present at any hour of the day or night), it
would have been a gift to have a caring individual stay with me at
night. We have created scads of matchmaking apps in the cyber
world; why can't we create something similar to match ICU and
other patients in need with trained and qualified loving, sensitive, caregiving volunteers, expanding on the ICU Hand-Holder
program I outlined in the previous chapter?

In my case, the hospital eventually splurged and hired a "sit-
ter" to watch me. This was not a compassionate move, however;
they merely caved to appease my distraught wife who learned

from a phone call that the one time she was not at my bedside, I nearly died due to negligence (recall my escape attempt and subsequent face plant). If a volunteer companion had been present when I was left alone that afternoon, I would not have been able to risk hurting myself by getting out of bed. As it was, I could have easily been more injured from hospital error than my actual trauma. After this episode, they did hire someone to look after me, but they also put me back in restraints, and so began the vicious cycle of stripping me of my humanity once again.

As a final note on bringing humanity into the ICU, I can attest that when medical personnel know something about the patient and his or her family, they are less likely to merely see a body and see a human being instead. Denise had the brilliant insight to know this, so she showed the ICU staff photographs of us and of our family. She knew it was crucial to humanize me so that the staff would think of me as a person; she wanted them to fight for me as much as she was. As I became weaker and my beard grew in gray, I looked like an old, cachectic man. To understand just how aged I looked, the first time the chief of trauma met Denise, he referred to me as her father, even though we are only five years apart. Looking the way I did on the outside, it would have been easy for the healthcare team to dismiss me as elderly, and even possibly deem me "expendable." But showing nurses photographs of our family together smiling, enjoying vacations and special events, put a human spin on me.

But what about when ICU patients are truly alone, with no family or friends to show these kinds of photos that humanize a virtual stranger to the hospital staff?

I propose an idea that my book collaborator, Stacey Aaronson, had that would not only "humanize" the ICU, but also give a more human connection to every patient.

Many facilities have a whiteboard for each patient where a

nurse writes relevant information. But the focus is on the medical—Who is the attending? Who is the nurse on shift?—not the patient. To bring the patient to the forefront, Stacey suggests adding a festive, artistic element that would both further humanize the patient *and* give a fun activity to the nurses who don't always have a lot of lighthearted moments in their work.

There are numerous vendors online that produce artistically made letters on heavy pressboard, the type that are used to create customized banners for various occasions by stringing the letters together. ICU wards could have an ample supply of the letters of the alphabet in bright colors (and I imagine generous donors would be happy to provide these to various hospitals if budget were an issue), and upon admission to the ICU, a patient's first name would be created with these letters and attached to the wall over his or her bed. But we would also take it an extra step: in addition to the individual letters for the names, there could be a supply of banners already made with the words "Grandma," "Grandpa," "Aunt," "Uncle," "Mama," "Papa," "Mr.," "Miss," etc. So someone named Millie might have "Grandma Millie" over her bed, or "Miss Millie," as people say in the South. In cases where the staff has no social information about the person, they can simply choose a title that feels appropriate and empowering, never derogatory. Every time a nurse or doctor approached a patient, they would see "Miss Millie" or "Grandpa Joe" or "Mama Rita" or "Mr. Daniel." They would then address the patient by this moniker, which would give a more personalized connection between staff and patient. It's much harder to dismiss a patient as a mere stranger when a familial nickname is attached to their first name—and the festive decor can only serve to make the ICU a friendlier, less maudlin place.

We make children's wards bright and pleasant. Why not the ICU?

◆

chapter twenty-seven

The Gravity of Maintaining HIPAA

After my fall, I was in an undeniably precarious situation. Not only did I have a bleed in my brain that could render me unable to work ever again, I was a patient in a trauma hospital where I once worked; there were physicians who provided care to me whom I knew personally, as well as physicians who were acquainted with people we knew in common. If any of those people leaked my condition such that it became public information, my practice could suffer—even if I made a completely full recovery, as fortunately I did.

This is precisely why the Health Insurance Portability and Accountability Act (HIPAA) was passed as a federal law in 1996, defining the proper management of protected health information (PHI), which is basically anything that can be used to identify an individual (name, address, even gender) linking them to diagnoses, diseases, allergies, etc.

All physicians are schooled on HIPAA, where it is emphasized that healthcare teams must not release identifiable information regarding patients unless specifically permitted. This extends even into the hallways of hospitals so that healthcare workers avoid speaking about a patient where others could accidentally overhear. For example, an innocent discussion between a physician and nurse in an elevator could unintentionally reveal PHI to the patient's neighbor, who happens to be in the elevator, visiting her mother on a different floor. Or a physician's office could accidentally release significant information regarding an adult child to her prying mother.

One would think that medical personnel would be religious about safeguarding patients' PHI, but the truth is, gossip is very difficult to quell, especially if it involves someone both people know. Even with reminders throughout hospitals, some with an index finger pushed against lips urging "ssssh," healthcare workers do not take this law seriously enough.

I found out just *how* irreverent people are to this law the day I returned to work.

At one of the hospitals where I attend—where none of the physicians work who administered to me during my trauma or the subsequent recovery—all of my colleagues should have been ignorant of the full extent of my injuries. The speed at which I returned should have had no bearing on *what* I had recovered from. In other words, these people saw me healthy several months prior, I was on a brief leave, and I was healthy when I returned. That scenario should have aroused no suspicion about how injured or ill I might have been. Again, no one should have been privy to *why* I was out, only *that* I was out. Yet the looks and comments of amazement I received that first day back painted a whole different story: my colleagues clearly knew how dire my situation had been; if they hadn't, there wouldn't have been such shock on their faces when they saw me.

Let me be clear: my wife and children told no one connected to me in the medical community of my extensive injuries, only basic minimal facts to justify my absence. My parents didn't tell my own family, let alone divulge my situation to any of their colleagues. The only people who knew intimate details were the doctors, nurses, and technicians who delivered care to me. I will never know how this private information became public.

While my Stoic philosophy keeps me from wasting anger toward the perpetrators, I was admittedly—and rightfully—devastated that people I trust and respect violated one of the primary tenets of our profession. The fact that they couldn't help themselves from discussing my status as a patient, knowing they could potentially ruin my reputation, and indeed my entire career, is deplorable. I even discovered that an operating-room technician knew confidential details about my clavicle fracture, though at no time did this information become public. Even worse, he proceeded to update the entire OR about my overall condition. Inaccurate rumors of an arm injury could have devastated my practice as a surgeon, yet the rumors flew nonetheless.

The other huge problem we must address is electronic medical records (EMR). Patients have little understanding how grossly these threaten our privacy. While having all their information in one centralized location has huge advantages, it also means that anyone at any time could learn a patient's most personal secrets. It also means that errors can easily propagate and auto-populate, as humans strangely have blind faith in computers.

Let me offer a perfect example.

I recently went to a new gastroenterologist for a routine colonoscopy. When I checked in, his medical assistant was reviewing my medications. Note that this physician's medical practice is not associated with either the trauma hospital or the rehabilitation facility where I was a patient. Yet the medical assistant began asking about a list of medications on my EMR that dated from my hospitalization four months prior. Somehow, many of the medications—all of which were stopped months before and some of which I had never even taken—were listed. When I told him I wasn't taking any of them, he was in disbelief. Clearly, his faith in the computer was greater than his faith in me, despite my being a physician. A simple push of the wrong button and these erroneous medications would have been renewed for me at the local pharmacy.

How did this happen?

To be honest, there could be several culprits.

The trauma hospital uses one system whereas the rehabilitation facility uses a different system. This particular GI practice happens to use the same system as the rehab facility. References to other physician visits showed up on my EMR, even though these practices don't use electronic medical records whatsoever. I can only imagine that somehow, there are multiple crossovers of data, including information that could be culled from insurance claims or pharmacy orders.

Nearly ten months after my trauma, when I saw another physician for a tracheostomy follow-up, his medical assistant named off the exact same erroneous list of medications from my ICU stay that the GI office had. I was shocked, as I had corrected that information with the assistant in that GI office months before. Plus, Denise and I are extraordinarily careful about not allowing release of any information. In fact, I always ask for my files to be locked; I am promised they are, yet I'm convinced it's not true.

What's clear is that the best EMR in the world cannot make up for human nature ot human error. And to make matters more terrifying, tech companies see EMR as the new data frontier—and this data can be leveraged. Simply Google "Project Nightingale." I can assure you this is not "fake news."

Another example is how HIPAA is frequently violated by healthcare workers when a celebrity is hospitalized—despite the fact that hospitals make a point of policing EMR access and firing employees who inappropriately view the EMR when a celebrity is admitted. Imagine how little oversight—whether from lack of staffing or lack of caring—goes into policing inappropriate access to the EMR for non-celebrities. As such, I have no way of feeling confident that if a colleague of mine wished to know the severity of my injuries, he or she could not easily access that data without repercussions. Since there are no "EMR police," perhaps it has already been done.

Another problem with an EMR is the actual protection of the database. An EMR used by wound care centers nationwide was recently hacked and access was lost for over a week. Although the firm guaranteed no data was breeched, there is so little controlling authority that it begs the question: How can anyone feel confident that this is true, when the security of our PHI is controlled by private industry focused on profit? It is only a matter of time before hackers hold PHI hostage for ransom. In fact, this has already happened in northern New Jersey at a major facility, yet it barely made the local news. The significance of this breech was tremendous, but after the ransom was paid and everything returned to "normal," there was no reaction of which I am aware. To me, this is foreshadowing that if we continue as we are, someone with a disease, such as HIV, who wishes to keep it confidential may be forced to pay people in Eastern Europe a king's ransom to prevent that information from being released to a list serve, or any other similar scenario.

While I don't want to end this chapter on a grim note, I want to emphasize that this is yet another area where we must be diligent about change. With all the brilliant minds creating these technologies, surely there are safeguards and methods that can be put into place to avoid unnecessary crossover between programs, information leaks, and erroneous reporting. Furthermore, there must be enforcement of these rules with real penalties. Lives of people can be destroyed when PHI is released. We must therefore not allow the foxes to guard the hen house. As someone who had chickens in his backyard, I can personally attest to how it does not end well for anyone.

When it comes to willful sharing of information between colleagues and others, there is simply no excuse for disregarding HIPAA. As professionals, we must be constantly self-aware of where, how loud, and to whom we speak, knowing that an innocent release of PHI can have severe consequences for any patient. Yes, we physicians are human, but what we may think is entertaining to share among ourselves about our patients completely violates their privacy, not to mention opens the door to obliterate someone's career, medical or otherwise.

Although I have been back to work for many months now, and one may say that none of this gossip hurt me in the long run, that isn't actually true. I had plenty of mountains to climb in my recovery alone, but the indiscriminate comments made in my professional circle definitely added further hurdles for me to clear. Had everyone with access to my private medical condition honored that my health situation was mine to discuss with only the people I chose, no one else's—just as every patient's health situation is theirs alone to share—I would have had a much smoother slide back into my work as surgeon. This is precisely what HIPAA is in place to protect, and is certainly every patient's right.

chapter twenty-eight

◆

The Necessity of
Insurance and Tort Reform

Whether or not you follow American politics, where a
great deal of emphasis has been placed on this topic
of late, you are likely painfully aware that our current system of
medical insurance is screaming for a major overhaul. And
though less discussed in public forums, medical litigation de-
mands an equal overhaul. This chapter aims to bring these issues
to light in a very personal way as part of my sweeping call for
massive change.

INSURANCE REFORM

Currently, I am insured through Denise's job, which carries a
typical deductible and out-of-pocket maximum. Unlucky for
us, since I was injured in late December, we hit the deductible
costs twice—once in 2018, and again in early 2019. Why so
close together, even though I never left the hospital? A matter
of only nine days meant the difference of thousands of dollars
out of my savings, because as you may be aware from your own
experience, despite the fact that accidents don't follow a calendar, out-of-pocket expenses reset in the new calendar year.

While we were fortunate to have savings to cover both deductibles, statistics show that the majority of Americans

wouldn't be able to afford a mere $400 hit in a single month. Had this been our situation, what would have happened?

Here is how the law currently stands:

> Since 1986, the Emergency Medical Treatment and Labor Act (EMTALA) has required all hospitals that accept Medicare (which is virtually all hospitals in the US) to provide screening and stabilization services to any patients who arrive in the emergency room, including women in active labor, regardless of the patient's insurance status or ability to pay for care.

This means the emergency room is required to screen all patients to determine what the problem is, and to provide stabilization services—they can't let a patient bleed to death on the floor because of a lack of funds. Courts have broadly expanded the definition of stabilizing care during emergencies so that doctors and hospitals are appropriately fearful of abandoning patients regardless of ability to pay. On the one hand, this is a good thing. But it also means the burden of paying for the uninsured is silently shifted to the insured. Add to this the need for many hospitals to generate large profits for multiple reasons, there is now even more pressure heaped on those with insurance to keep the system afloat.

Perhaps we have not really addressed the root cause, because although the Affordable Care Act from 2010 was supposed to have addressed this, it essentially only expanded Medicaid and put into place stringent metrics to claw back payments. In short, it has made things arguably worse.

In my case, for just one example, what would have become of me if we couldn't afford our deductible despite having insurance? In the midst of the scariest, most stressful time in

Denise's life, she would have been faced with negotiating a payment plan, taking an early distribution from retirement (which takes time to process), selling some of our things for extra money, or asking others for help. Who wants to be worried about meeting a deductible through these means when a spouse is fighting for his or her life—and whose further care may in fact be delayed because a deductible hasn't yet been paid? And I won't even touch what happens to the disadvantaged people who are completely alone and in this predicament. I'm sure you can guess what level of care—and how much of it—they typically receive.

The bigger issue is, even when patients *can* make their deductible, the under-insured, or those simply responsible for the portion insurance doesn't pay, can be financially wiped out by a trauma such as mine. Due to the way our system performs accounting to maximize collections, costs are horribly inflated for everything from an IV to a feeding tube to a major surgery; with every medical intervention, every piece of equipment, every consult, I could not help but think of the additional costs accrued. And with good reason:

To date, the charges submitted for my care easily exceed $1,000,000.

You read that right: *one million dollars.*

Even more bizarre is that although bills were submitted, because many of the providers and facilities were in-network, the charges were adjusted through contracts and the payouts were much less. The reason for this rests in our uniquely American system of healthcare finance.

When insurance companies came into existence, they contracted with many (not all) providers. When a contract exists between an insurance carrier and a provider or facility, that relationship is considered in-network. Once in-network, the charges (or bills) are renegotiated to in-network rates, which are presumably reasonable. However, the charges themselves remain inflated so as to maximize collections from patients who have out-of-network insurance, or no insurance at all. This system also allows providers and facilities to negotiate higher rates by claiming they are heavily discounted.

If this sounds like madness, it is. In fact, it is no different from this simple analogy:

Imagine buying dinner in a restaurant where the costs are significantly reduced from those advertised because you belong to a certain club. While you pay a much lesser price, the couple next to you pays an inflated price because they don't belong to the club. To add to the disparity, the prices are not clearly posted on the menu, and the bill is presented only after ordering. Crazy, right?

That's precisely how our current insurance system operates.

While private insurance plans vary quite a bit based on what people can afford for premiums, it is common for patients to be left with a *minimum* of 20% of their total *allowable* medical bill. In my case, that would equal at least $200,000, if it were all out-of-network. Even with a payment plan, the vast majority could never afford such a high extra monthly expense, not to mention the years of accrued interest it would require to pay it off. Why the system is set up in this fashion makes little sense. Almost no one could survive paying these bills directly.

Even the marketplace for purchasing plans makes little sense. Since our nation has evolved into employers providing the healthcare plan, cost-cutting is rampant and the rules vary from state to state. And what if you're an individual or entrepreneur who wishes to purchase his or her own plan? You're faced with grossly expensive options or inadequate plans that cover next to nothing. There must be a level of patient obligation to prevent people from over-utilizing care, but the rising deductibles for the masses are unconscionable. A cursory glance may suggest that a one-payor system like Medicare may indeed solve many of the problems, but the question is: can our country truly afford it? And make no mistake that a one-payer system may metamorphose into a Medicaid-like scheme where quality simply lacks. Rationing will also take place, as costs would be prohibitive. Since most patients are too injured to survive chest wall plating, for one example, I can only imagine what would have happened to me.

ANOTHER FORM OF corruption within our current system is commercial insurance companies playing tricks on the insured to dodge claims. This speaks to profit motive.

Rather than use a global occurrence, our insurance company required us to file a specific accident form for each provider claim—in other words, a certain form must literally be linked to each individual claim. You might imagine how confusing this can become, and I would go so far as to say that this is the insurance company's goal. They so desperately seek to avoid responsibility of payment that they create a virtual web of forms and caveats that confounds even the most intelligent person. In our case, they would respond to the billing entity that we—the patient and family—were sent an accident form but did not return it. These forms were not only infrequently sent to us, but when they were, the forms came weeks after the insurance company had already denied the claim due to an absent form. When these providers were faced with a claim "denial," they started to bill us. And these bills were outrageously high, because the providers would charge whatever they wanted without the in-network insurance company adjusting their fees.

Why is this possible when a person has insurance?

Because even though a provider may be in-network with the plan, once a claim is denied, many providers simply bill the patient whatever amount they wish.

Imagine the diligence with which Denise had to go over these charges and claims, all while being my advocate in the hospital, all day, every day. Thank goodness she had the smarts and wherewithal to call the insurance company and fight their strategy. But this is what that fight looked like for her:

She had to link every submitted charge to a specific accident form, then demand that the insurance company reprocess each claim.

Meanwhile, she had to call every provider to doggedly ensure they knew she was working on their claims so that we would not be sent to collections.

She had to make sure the staff in accounts receivable switched our balances from patient responsibility back to insurance.

Eventually, *months later*, the claims processed.

Yes, we were still hit with high deductibles and co-payments, but at least the claims finally went through.

Can you imagine if a patient didn't have a spouse or loved one? I would never have been able to handle this feat on my own; I was too focused on rebuilding my strength and returning to my life to even attempt navigating such a maze. I'm not exaggerating when I say it's clear that the system is rigged to put the onus on the individual, since the individual holds little or no power to fight back. Families are frequently torn apart— after having survived a nightmare—when the bills come in. If my family, with my MD and Denise's MBA, had to struggle, I shudder to think how difficult it is for scores of families across America.

Once I was in rehab, new insurance struggles arose. For example, by contract, I was entitled to a maximum of only 35 outpatient physical therapy sessions. That may seem like a lot, but I wanted and needed more. As a physician, when I ran out of visits, I could perform my own therapy, but it certainly was not the same. In cases like mine, that maximum was simply not enough after a catastrophic fall. Where is the plan that has a contingency for situations like this?

THE SUBJECT I broach, and the question we must pose is: How can physicians advocate in the best interests of their patients if they are no longer independent agents?

As I just eluded above, here's a bit more history to explain what I mean.

Back when physicians were paid directly by patients in the early twentieth century, or through a third-party insurance company in the second half of the same century, doctors could order tests and make recommendations centered on the specific issues affecting the patient. But, as is human nature, prices kept escalating. Was it greed? Was it inflation? Was it the golden goose? Who knows?

To cap the out-of-control pricing, government created Medicare and Medicaid as a safety net for the elderly and poor. Meanwhile, the free market created commercial health insurance companies that more aggressively managed the physicians. It seemed like a brilliant solution, but unfortunately, all this did was move the flow of money to a new source: many insurance companies are no longer patient-focused and are instead geared toward maximizing profit. By making physicians follow what is called "population healthcare," we are forced to ascribe to the philosophy that the needs of the many outweigh the needs of the few. But on an individual basis, this protocol may negatively impact, or even lead to the death, of a patient.

For example, if you are the one who has a missed metastatic lesion because a scan was considered unnecessary by an insurance company, you have been failed 100 percent by the system. I live this every day when I treat my patients with malignant melanoma. I know that a PET scan can detect metastatic lesions or second primaries, and to date, I have saved five patient lives because I ordered PET scans in low-risk patients. The rub is, insurance companies actively discourage these scans, considering them unnecessary because of the cost-to-benefit ratio. Even Medicare negatively scores me for over-utilizing this technology. This is just one example of how profit translates into missed opportunities for patients—a missed opportunity being another phrase for "a life saved."

As a practicing surgeon, I see insurance companies purposely making payment for service more difficult by increasing the requirements for providers to receive payments. The audit frequency has increased dramatically. This delays payment and many times allows the company to simply not pay a claim because a "t" is not crossed or an "i" is not dotted. The denials for services rendered have increased to an unbearable level for physicians, hospitals, and patients. It goes without saying that all of these strategies maximize profits, not deliver healthcare.

I offer a recent specific example.

I was called by an insurance company to see if I would consider performing a procedure in a surgical center rather than a hospital—presumably because the surgical center is less costly than the hospital for the insurance company. The procedure, known as a sentinel lymph node biopsy, involves the injection of radioactive tracer dye at the skin site of a melanoma, after which the surgeon locates the now radioactive lymph node that drains that specific region of skin. It is an amazing technology that allows early metastatic disease to be detected. I explained to the representative that these dyes are typically injected in the hospital due to the regulatory costs of managing the radioactive tracer, and that after it is injected, I have 12 to 18 hours before the tracer dissipates. He suggested I have the patient travel to the surgical center from the hospital after the injection, which is logistically doable but certainly not convenient (or arguably safe) for the patient.

Meanwhile, I asked who would pay for the probe I needed to perform the procedure, which is essentially a Geiger counter, to locate the lymph node. (I happen to know it costs $14,000, as my surgical team accidentally discarded one such probe that had to be replaced.) He informed me that entrepreneurial surgeons were already doing these procedures at surgical centers, perhaps with personal financial benefit in saving the insurance company from the higher cost associated at the hospital. I immediately saw how surgeons could be motivated by profit-sharing with the surgical center, and that insurance companies would perhaps pay the surgeon more when procedures were performed at a desired location. Ultimately, the representative warned me the insurance company would soon no longer pay for these procedures to be performed in the hospital as they were too expensive. I was crestfallen that yet another roadblock was being placed in front of me to perform a procedure that could potentially save a person's life, not to mention we must support safe and well-performing hospitals, as those are where lives are saved.

Insurance companies are also denying authorizations for surgery more often. When a medical director examines pictures and decides whether he or she will authorize a surgery, we have companies literally practicing medicine without a license. For example, I had a patient with a mole on her lip who complained that it felt like it was burning. Although benign, this was an indication to remove it. (Medicine even has a term to describe this phenomenon: it's called "inflamed.") Nevertheless, the company, in its pursuit of maximizing profit, called the procedure cosmetic and refused to cover it. Despite my holding a 12-minute conversation with the reviewer, we had no choice but to cancel the procedure. What was most egregious was that the representative ended the call by saying she was not dictating medical care, and that I should do what I think is the right action. Of course, if I went ahead with "doing what is right," I wouldn't get paid for it, and the patient would be stuck with a bill, even though she pays insurance premiums from her salary.

Another increasing event is the denial of services rendered.

Surgeons have codes created by the American Medical Association for each maneuver they perform, and guidelines exist regarding their usage. Every surgery requires an operative report, where the surgeon describes the procedure performed for medicolegal reasons and links the procedure to codes for billing purposes. However, the insurance companies will frequently audit these reports using their own coding interpretation rather than the ones established. In other words, the companies will often deny services, stating the report does not match the coding. Appeals are generally useless. Why? Because the people interpreting the coding are either directly employed or engaged by the insurance company. Not only do the appeals take months but there is infrequently an independent review board.

Meanwhile, the CEOs of these companies, after exercising stock options, often earn more than 40 million dollars per year. You read that correctly. This is money that could save lives or allow improved quality for hundreds if not thousands of customers, but instead it is in the pockets of the captains of this industry. Where are the voices asking just how much is enough? Shouldn't the same morality I ask of healthcare workers apply to the entire industry?

Unfortunately, predatory physicians are part of the problem as well—something toward which the medical world seems to turn a blind eye. For example, as a physician, I know how to code for an in-patient hospital consultation, yet in reviewing my medical bills from my trauma, I witnessed over-coding performed by some physicians in order to inappropriately bill a higher level of care. I also saw out-of-network billing at elevated rates for which there was no transparency. One of my surgeons actually received $30,000 from insurance. No one physician is worth being paid the cost of a new car for an afternoon's work.

I am grateful to be alive, but there is something terribly wrong with our reimbursement system.

AS YOU MIGHT imagine, all of these competing and indeed debilitating factors are nearly enough to make a physician consider leaving medicine. But perhaps the most egregious problem occurs when physicians are directly employed by a healthcare system, as they are pushed hard to make patient referrals to specific facilities or other hired individuals, increasing profits at the potential cost of quality. This abuse was highlighted in a 2019 article in *The Atlantic*[2], citing that when Dr. Susan Youngs had concerns that a Michigan doctor was inappropriately reading studies to maximize profit, she was simply ignored. This is shocking and unconscionable, yet it is also increasingly commonplace.

---

[2] Khazan, Olga. "Why Some Doctors Purposely Misdiagnose Patients." *The Atlantic.* Aug 15, 2019.

All of this corruption has led to patients having to be wary of where they are referred. In the past, independent physicians would refer patients to whomever they believed were most qualified to treat the illness. Now, many physicians will only send patients to colleagues within their own system to maximize profit. This current system of "super-groups" is geared toward maximizing revenue for the company, not delivering the best in patient care. And when you add the sizable amount of money put toward advertising and marketing, facilities are literally fighting each other for patients instead of fighting disease.

To make it worse, physicians are under pressure—and many times even tracked—to keep patients within their system. Think of it like team sports, where physicians wear a t-shirt of a specific color and send patients only to those physicians who wear the same color. In doing so, they maximize revenue for the "team." In the same way, physicians may bring patients to a certain facility based on their personal ownership rather than quality. As you can imagine, this is incredibly divisive—it is truly not so different from having scads of sports teams in competition with each other, and each of those teams having a legion of fans. This may be fine in the athletic arena, but medicine is not a sport, and it certainly should not be divided up into teams that deem ability much less important than the "employer" who has the best funding.

AS OUR SYSTEM exists currently, the entire in- versus out-of-network system is an insane maze. Although New Jersey law now requires that out-of-network physicians identify themselves prior to delivering non-emergent care, not one of my providers who were out-of-network identified themselves as such. Remember the psychologist at the rehab facility? This

meant we were subject to much higher billing for these procedures—and these out-of-network charges border on criminally
expensive. Why is the drive for this over-billing so pervasive?

While there are certainly physicians who are mired in the
prestige of their position and drawn to it affording them a luxurious lifestyle, the truth is that it is extremely costly to fund a
medical practice: extensive office computer systems, high rent,
medical malpractice insurance and claims, staff salaries, to list
but a few. This is why organizations have been so successful in
buying physicians' practices and then directing patient volume
to themselves. Unfortunately, all of this results in socking the
patients with huge bills.

HOW DO WE break this concerning trend of insurance companies "owning" the field of medicine for their own personal
gain? Clearly market forces alone are inadequate, as this is how
we got into this mess.

I propose that we return physicians to independent status.

Now, you may be thinking, isn't that what got us into the
exact same scenario that insurance companies were supposed
to solve? Yes. But recall that mess was created by those who
abandoned their Hippocratic Oath. Sadly, such physicians still
exist, and they've even been assisted in their greed by the systems in place. In an ideal world, this would never be an issue in
medicine. But since we can't always rely on an individual's
ethics, we would need measures in place to monitor and disal-
low overpricing of procedures. We would once again have to
call on the brilliant minds in our community to craft this new
system, but once in place, we as physicians could once again be
able to advocate solely for our patients and minimize competing conflicts of interest.

One such option is to return to medical payment as it was

in the 1960s but add our current level of technology. Here's how this might look:

All procedures would have a nationally recognized, reasonable cost that would be published and accessible to all patients on the internet. Since we are not a communist society, no provider is required to charge these rates. However, for each procedure, individual doctors would be required to list their prices as well. For example, a specific procedure may have a nationally recognized cost of $1,000, but Dr. Jones might charge $5,000 and Dr. Smith may charge $500. Patients would then be able to shop and compare, just as they do for nearly every other item in our free market. The same pricing system would be true for hospitals. Instead of charging inflated rates as they do today to maximize insurance payments, there would be more competitive pricing. Emergency care would follow the same model, but we would establish a maximum national standard for urgent procedures performed while physicians were on-call. In other words, an urgent appendectomy performed by a surgeon who charges twice the national average could be multiplied by 15% for urgency, but no more. This transparency would allow patients to shop for an elective hysterectomy no differently than how they shop for a refrigerator.

You may be asking, then, how would insurance work? The short answer is, much better. There would be a smorgasbord of policies available in the free-market system. Young healthy individuals could elect to buy inexpensive policies for catastrophic coverage only. Or, if they were so inclined, a moderate policy would reimburse up to several times the reasonable costs, whereas a Cadillac policy would cover a much higher factor. Medicaid would be a safety net only for those who cannot afford care, and it would adhere to the same reimbursement rates for procedures so that patients could shop for providers. Medicare, too, would exist as it does now for those disabled or 65 years and older. Meanwhile, the financing of this would actually be more predictable, as all costs would be transparent.

Note that it would be incumbent on physicians to keep an eye on pricing, as market forces would truly be at work. Hence, medical staffs would police themselves, keeping all physicians accountable and voting those who charge outrageous amounts off the medical staff. For the skeptical, doctors could not price fix, for the same reasons it is currently illegal in retail.

This proposal demonstrates that we must rebuild our broken system in an entirely new fashion. Doing that means introducing something never done before.

In sum, the notion of a patient's "value"—and therefore their care—being dependent upon their insurance plan, or if their deductible is met, is unconscionable. And the common practice of overcharging that occurs every day in our country, at the expense of individuals in need of vital medical care, demonstrates the further downward spiral of our current system. Whether that can be solved through a variation of the above scenario, Medicare for all, or some other form of universal healthcare remains to be seen. But one thing is for certain: in our current system, not everyone is receiving the care they need, and we do not have enough funds to maintain what we currently have in place. Therefore, everyone is destined to lose.

TORT REFORM

Though I'm merely scratching the surface of this topic here, no conversation about healthcare would be complete without discussion of tort reform.

In today's society, physicians are forced to constantly think about the possibility of being sued. There are certainly cases of gross negligence—amputation of the wrong limb, surgeons performing procedures solely for money that they're not actually qualified to do, and other unacceptable situations—but they are thankfully the exception rather than the norm. Yet when complications from procedures and surgeries *do* occur, even though the risks are clearly spelled out to patients and they must give their written consent, our cultural norms encourage people to demand compensation even if negligence was *not* a factor. It is as if we expect the perfect *outcome* to be the standard of care rather than the perfect *process*, which is simply not possible.

This fear of litigation leads to over-prescription as a safety net. For example, I have seen antibiotics given when a "watch and wait" approach would have been equally appropriate. But if antibiotics *aren't* given, and a condition such as cellulitis of the leg turns into an abscess, not only will that doctor worry about litigation, but you can rest assured the patient will leave a scathing review on the internet—*and* consider suing the physician. Hence, prescribing the antibiotic gives everyone peace of mind, whether or not it is truly justified. A deleterious result of this, however, is that antibiotic-resistant infections are becoming a major global problem.

Anytime a patient requires medical attention—or seeks intervention of some kind voluntarily—there is the risk of human error. While no doctor ever wants to make a critical mistake with a patient, the fact that we *are* human means we cannot be infallible, no matter how hard we may try. Further, any misstep (which is nearly always unintentional), can land us in a lawsuit that could cripple or obliterate our ability to practice. In short, the pressure to deliver impeccable results (outcome) at all times is enormous, despite following processes that meet the standard of care.

The good news for physicians who are truly victims of meritless patient claims is that most medical malpractice cases do not make it to trial—and even fewer win for the plaintiff. However, although the system works objectively by filtering out frivolous claims, the monetary and emotional costs to doctors are astronomical. And because we don't currently have a national standard in place for these cases, blatant subjectivity exists. Court venues play a role; certain counties in the US are consistently friendlier to plaintiffs. This is why I call for establishing a national model that will put this subjectivity to rest.

What might that look like?

On a base level, I propose that medical panels comprised of trained experts and laypeople set a national standard, with well-defined awards in the cases of negligence, as caps on awards have shown to limit outrageous jury actions. Though I realize this will require some thoughtful deliberation on the part of these panels, there are certainly enough brilliant minds in our community to come to a solution that would go a long way in helping to protect both physicians and patients within the legal arena. In fact, we have already seen evidence of this in the state of Texas.

WHEN IT COMES to health insurance and tort reform, there's no doubt we have a substantial journey ahead, one that is sure to be fraught with differing opinions. But simply because something may seem daunting does not mean we should merely avoid it for another decade or more. None of it will change if we as patients *and* physicians don't make our voices heard against these corrupt and grossly imbalanced systems in place today. Everyone in our country deserves so much better, and I sincerely believe that together we can make the kind of sweeping transformation necessary in these areas for the greater good of all of us.

◆

chapter twenty-nine

Taking a Closer Look at
Disability Coverage

As a solo practitioner of medicine, I work for myself. This means that if I don't work, there is no money coming in. Until my trauma, I'd never been faced with a prolonged absence from my practice. But after being in the daunting position of having no earnings flowing in, I understand just how crucial it is to have disability coverage.

I also now understand how tempting it might be for some people to stay on it long term, and why it is often abused.

Trauma carries with it financial ramifications as well as emotional and physical ones. I had no one to blame but myself for my fall, and I certainly couldn't sue my homeowner's insurance, or the ladder company, or even my roof. So the fact that I had paid into a personally funded disability policy was a relief—until Denise discovered just what a hassle it was to obtain the benefits.

After my fall, she managed to find a statement for my policy, and although it was a pathetically inadequate amount, it was certainly better than nothing. But when she called to inquire about receiving the benefit, they refused to speak with her unless she had a power of attorney statement. You may recall in an earlier chapter that obtaining this required two full days of Denise filling out maddening paperwork and having several phone calls with our attorney. Once she had all the proper documents in place, she thought it would be smooth sailing for the disability payout. But she was wrong.

Adding even more to her stress level, the disability company required a heap of additional paperwork. Finding these numerous documents, from tax statements to office billing records, was a colossal task. She then had to submit these and follow up—all while staying at my bedside the entire day. She had to go through a similar bureaucratic web at our local bank in order to gain control of my business finances. When all of that was accomplished, it turned out that my 22 years of payments for disability insurance added up to more than what I received in benefits. Clearly, I was left to question the merit of the type of insurance I'd invested in.

For many people, however, disability policies pay out as long as you are deemed disabled, until age 65. Mine wasn't set up that way, but I can imagine how, when someone has been through a devastating accident or illness, it might be an attractive option to continue receiving those benefits, even after the person has recovered and is not technically "disabled" anymore. For the same reasons people try to sue someone after an injury for remuneration, if this payout actually compensates for a person not working, or provides enough to help a family who is struggling, it can be a benefit that's difficult to let go.

Therein lies the abuse of the system.

For me, the financial pressure of not having enough disability to support us was a motivator to return to work as rapidly as possible. But as a physician, I've witnessed patients continue to experience symptoms solely because they have secondary gain. In other words, if they're still "sick," they can justify missing work or receiving disability payments. I know this sounds harsh, but it's unfortunately a reality. Of course, severely injured people deserve disability. But if someone has recovered well, and all signs point to that being the case, I ask that we as physicians scrutinize these forms more closely that document limitations (and I further suggest that we need some form of legal protection from the angry patient we may have just informed that we can no longer sign off on their disability forms).

I am amazed by the number of people who remain on Medicare disability after near complete resolution of their symptoms. For morbid obesity alone, I have multiple examples of patients who are on disability. After undergoing successful bariatric surgery and losing more than 100 pounds, these patients develop a pannus (loose skin of the abdomen) that hangs so low they cannot walk. After I perform surgery to remove the pannus, they are able to walk without difficulty and are essentially cured. Yet some of these patients still receive disability. This apparently occurs because there is no formal review process to re-evaluate the need for permanent benefits, or if there is, it is certainly broken. I have filed paperwork for both short- and long-term benefits for patients, but never once have I been contacted to reassess the status of a disabled patient. In my case, without substantial disability insurance benefits available, I had no choice but to return to work as soon as possible.

As I can attest, it is frightening to go through a trauma and to know that on top of what you're facing physically and emotionally, a halted income looms large too. A loss in earnings, as well as large medical expenses, can be itemized and filed at tax time. But what about the money needed to fill the gas tank or pay the rent? For this reason, I propose a re-envisioning of how our disability system works, not only for the traditionally employed, but also for solo practitioners as well as the unemployed.

In the face of true tragedy, we would do well as a nation to lessen the burden of zero incoming wages from an injured person's and family's long list of concerns. We have worker's compensation for work-related injuries, but did you know it doesn't kick in for an employer, only an employee? If the employer is blessed, he or she may have enough savings to survive, but what if that's not the case? And what about completely innocent accidents not related to work? There are charities for injured police, firefighters, and the military. But what about the self-employed who are the backbone of our economy?

Why can't we as a nation offer low-interest, easy-to-obtain disability loans to those needing coverage during a time of crisis, similar to how we offer loans to students for their education? Student loans have become a massive burden on our young people, and we certainly need a major re-evaluation of student loan forgiveness, but as with so many proposals I've made in this book, we possess numerous intelligent thinkers who are capable of improving this system. Imagine what a relief it could be for an individual or a family to know there were funds readily available to help them survive a time of crisis. Qualifying would only require a physician's signature and the filling out of a simple form, not piles of paperwork and tax statements. And with it being a loan, not a gift, people would be motivated to return to work, and not as likely to squander the funds.

Of course, as with any revamp within our medical system, we must be cognizant of how a new vision of disability insurance could be abused and build in a method of checks and balances. But I know I'm not alone when I say that our citizens could certainly use, and would deeply appreciate, monetary assistance during a time when all hope can very well seem lost.

◆

chapter thirty

The Egregious Nature of
Profit-Driven Healthcare—
and What Our Country Needs Instead

I spent much of Chapter Twenty-Eight describing a healthcare financial system that remains mostly capitalistic and is subject to market forces. While I am not a socialist, I admit I am grappling with proposing a moral solution. Having said that, let us look at some of the healthcare systems on our globe.

As a volunteer surgeon, I am needed most in underdeveloped countries. Most of these countries where I have often worked, such as Nepal or Guatemala, have private and public medicine existing side by side. The private system functions no differently than the unadulterated free market. Unfortunately, that means prices are exorbitant for much of the indigent population. Furthermore, price gouging occurs. Meanwhile, the sanctioned government hospitals only provide minimal care of poor quality. And while the pharmacies offer many drugs at significantly lower prices than in the US, some of these medications are pirated and of questionable quality, whereas others are indeed packaged identically to those in our country. Clearly, this is not ideal, but given the poor economies of these countries, this is the best they can offer to cover the greatest number of souls.

On the other hand, many advanced nations, such as Israel

and Canada, have a system wherein people have access to truly outstanding care that is covered by the government. There is significant rationing and there are long waits, but there is government coverage nonetheless. Medications are indeed reasonably priced, but not all prescribed products are available as they are in the US.

In the United States, we arguably have an amazing array of treatments available but at an astronomical cost. So much of our economy is wrapped up in healthcare that we have multiple parties trying to guarantee a livelihood. It seems as if our country wants their cake and to eat it too.

Let's look at my personal experience with a near life-ending event.

The trauma surgeon who saved my life was remarkable. Not only was he a skilled surgeon, but he was instilled with a moral code exemplified by his two tours of duty with the US Army. He was also a physician employed directly by his hospital. In fact, all of the physicians who treated me were from this same system.

The system that ultimately saved my life was a charity hospital, one initially created with a strong religious foundation whose mission was clear to everyone: placing the patient at the center. I've outlined in this book multiple ways that I felt failed by the hospital, but here I want to be clear that it wasn't necessarily the *hospital* itself that failed me, but rather the prevalent *system* within which most hospitals operate in our country today that influenced much of the treatment I received—both beneficial and detrimental, life-saving and life-altering. It is precisely the for-profit model of healthcare delivery that I believe may be the root cause of our failing system, as even many nonprofit systems are now pushing hard to make significant money. This must be put under a microscope if we hope to make meaningful change in the medical community, and this is why it is the topic of my final chapter.

LET'S START BY going back in time and taking a look at the Wild West in the US. In the 1800s, anyone could sell anything and call it a curative elixir. Before the 1910 Flexner Report (named after educator Abraham Flexner from Kentucky, who went on to establish the Institute for Advanced Study in Princeton, New Jersey) that revolutionized medical training and was published by the Carnegie Foundation, anyone could call themselves a physician with any type of apprenticeship. (Note, however, that while Flexner helped to streamline medical schools, he also deemed the natural healing modalities that had existed for hundreds of years quackery, hence the beginning of pharmaceutical medicine over holistic, and the eschewing of the importance of nutrition on a person's well-being, both of which have had massive negative repercussions on society.)

It has now been over a century since an independent academic like Flexner has analyzed our medical education system from top to bottom. Meanwhile, there has never been an academic report addressing our healthcare delivery system in a similar manner of which I am aware. In other words, it is time for our society to demand another Flexner-style report that addresses these critical issues. We must look long and hard at how our capitalist society has led to our current healthcare system and how we can keep the positive aspects of it while recognizing that we must never compromise on quality in the name of profit. We must also compare it to the delivery systems of other economically advantaged countries, which begs the questions:

Can outstanding healthcare be delivered by a facility that is seeking to maximize profit?

Can a health insurance company that is geared toward increasing its quarterly shareholders' returns truly finance stellar care for people?

I was not only struggling just prior to my fall with the concept of how profit-driven healthcare has become a reality, but I was already convinced it was doing irreparable damage to our beloved field of medicine—both to the care-*givers* and to the care-*receivers*.

Why? There are several reasons.

CEOS AND HEALTHCARE ARE NOT APPROPRIATE PARTNERS

One problem with a for-profit hospital is that they are run by CEOs in a business-like fashion. By nature of the job, CEOs are tasked with placing profit above everything else. When high earnings are the primary mission, however, aggressive (and therefore successful) business leaders in healthcare conveniently forget that the final "product" they are aiming to produce is the extension of life. Nearly any shortcut that increases the bottom line directly hurts patient care; a human being may be maimed or not saved from dying so that the corporation can make more money.

Adding further insult is that many successful CEOs have narcissistic personalities. While this is certainly not true of all CEOs, it is nonetheless one of the qualities that often allows them to rise to their high position. Unfortunately, this is precisely the wrong quality for a patient-focused hospital. In other words, CEOs tend to be good business leaders for the *corporation* but terrible advocates for *patient care*.

Take, for example, that CEOs of for-profit hospitals frequently make light of the fact that from a tax viewpoint, their facility is no different from a Walmart or Staples, when in reality they should actually see their facility as more like a museum or a Goodwill store. They further state that although the tax status of the for-profit hospital may be different from other hospitals, the mission is not. This could not be further from the truth. The for-profit status literally means that any money made is distributed to investors, not reinvested into the community. Further, for-profit hospitals cannot maintain foundations, which are the backbone of community service and frequently provide money for improved equipment, elevated quality, and stellar nursing care. As a direct result of profit being handed to investors instead of reinvested into the community, this money is taxed by the government. Hence, for-profit healthcare is indeed treated no differently than any other commercial business from a tax standpoint.

Should healthcare be commoditized like a restaurant or a hotel?

Of course not.

Is this happening more and more throughout our country?

Sadly, yes.

To make matters worse, CEOs frequently promote only those people who share their vision of profit over patients. This means they surround themselves with "yes-ing" physicians who collaborate with them, and who directly benefit financially from maintaining silence about poor quality, ignoring their professional duty to protect patients from harm. It is not uncommon to see these CEOs, with only profits in mind, manipulate the medical staff bylaws for their advantage, and because of the hierarchy, the medical leadership can do very little to oppose it.

While it is illegal to pay physicians directly for referrals, there are gaping loopholes that are not adequately policed, allowing an incredible number of physicians to receive stipends from hospitals for essentially making referrals. One way this functions is that physicians are frequently named as "directors" of service lines and receive payments for performing oversight and maintaining quality. When I was in such a position, I naively poured hours of work every week into developing and growing programs with measurable successful outcomes. But once I began calling out deep quality issues and actively decreasing my volume at the facility when my concerns were ignored, I was "released" from my duties. The physicians who took over my former leadership roles had little, if any, experience or interest in these service lines—and everyone knew this was done merely so that they could receive a stipend, thereby buying referrals. The shame in all of this is that on a municipal or state level, there is simply too much work for inspectors to continually police hospitals for this practice. Meanwhile, some physicians log imaginary directorship hours without any legal consequence.

Again, business leaders tend to naturally focus on the financial mission—yet when business leaders who are CEOs of medical facilities do so, they seem to easily forget that patients are supposed to matter above all else. This shift in power that has occurred from physicians making critical decisions about resources in healthcare to businesspeople now making those decisions has undeniably taken medicine in a frightening, and sometimes deadly, direction.

Further, when hospital administration places their sole focus on making money, healthcare workers suffer too. It doesn't take long for hospital employees to realize that fulfilling their oaths to patients isn't valued by their employer, which leads to moral injury. They may continue to serve their patients from their own desire and commitment to deliver phenomenal care, but as many people can attest, that can be difficult to sustain when "the boss" doesn't appreciate or even encourage it. As I saw firsthand, both in the ICU and in rehab, many healthcare workers under those circumstances often lose their sense of caring and resort to merely "getting through" a shift or "servicing" patients instead of truly caring for them, not to mention the occurrence of sometimes fatal errors.

And you might imagine how these nurses and technicians feel forced to keep silent about problems when they witness what happens to those physicians who speak up. I have actually heard in boardroom discussions that in business terms, it is like shooting a hostage to show you are serious.

In our current environment, the reasons physicians are terrified to make their voices heard about safety are twofold: 1) physicians *not* employed by the hospital will lose critical referrals; and 2) physicians who *are* employed by the hospital risk being fired or marginalized if they speak up. There is no whistleblower protection for physicians in these situations, as those who complain about poor quality are subsequently accused of being disruptive. This is what happened to me. I now realize I could never singlehandedly effectuate positive change in such a climate.

LACK OF GOVERNMENT OVERSIGHT AND NATIONAL STANDARDS NEGATIVELY IMPACT PATIENT CARE

One huge problem with for-profit healthcare is that there is no meaningful government oversight of the decision-making processes that directly affect patient care. That means if profits trump patients, no one is directly supervising this missive except for those who directly benefit from the profits.

We have unbiased LeapFrog surveys to grade hospital performance, but to rely solely on market forces to punish those facilities that perform poorly is inadequate. Unlike New York City restaurants that can lose their clientele to local competition when they receive a B or C grade by inspectors (see the ABCEats program of New York City), hospitals generally maintain a monopoly in the region they serve. In other words, it may not be prudent for a patient to travel to another hospital to avoid the low-grade one; hence, the hospital leans on these "guaranteed" patients in the "catchment area" (a real term used) who may not have any better option, despite the poor-quality care patients receive there.

You may be wondering, what about smaller hospitals that don't have a monopoly?

Hospitals are now rushing to join what are called unified systems. In these situations, smaller hospitals serve as feeders for the bigger "mothership" hospital—the one that has the established name and, in the best cases, the higher reputation. What this means is they can send someone to an "associated" hospital in the unified system—even if that smaller hospital has reported lapses in quality—and cash in on that connection. Furthermore, as hospitals consolidate into the same system, competition is further reduced, thereby increasing bargaining power. This is no different from a company such as Amazon gobbling up companies like Whole Foods. Whole Foods stores still operate, but they're now under the Amazon umbrella, and Amazon is the one who makes all the big decisions. These hospitals operate in much the same way.

How do we keep this parasitic-style monopolizing approach from growing?

One potential option is to establish strict government-regulated metrics for all hospitals, regardless of ownership, by those who best understand: the physicians, not the bureaucrats. These metrics would span the entire spectrum of the healthcare experience and be rigidly enforced nationwide; because state and/or municipal politics are too susceptible to straying from the mission, federal oversight would be required. Failure to meet any of these federalized requirements would not be accepted. Further, there would be no allowance for these infractions to be merely "worked on" in any situation that translates into patient falls, acquired infections, or even patient deaths from wrongly administered medications. In other words, the same way a restaurant is closed to preserve public health when it fails a Board of Health inspection, so too should a hospital. I think anyone would agree that the threat of closure is a much more powerful motivator than a slap on the hand that allows failing hospitals to continue risking the lives of patients.

But what if a hospital is doing poorly and is the only one in town? What is the local populace supposed to do if it closes?

At this point, I don't have a perfect answer for that unfortunate scenario. But what I will say is this:

Medical errors are commonly hidden by facilities for fear of litigation; transparency translates into severe financial losses. This means that patients remain ignorant of the facts and are robbed of the opportunity to educate themselves about quality of care. The idea that people with only one local hospital would choose it blindly, completely unaware of how poor the care was, demonstrates a huge lapse in medical ethics. Additionally, these facilities cannot improve flawed processes by learning from their errors if they do not acknowledge these errors exist.

For example, it appears a much greater percentage of for-profit hospitals repeatedly score poorer over time on the Leapfrog Group safety grade than the nonprofit hospitals. As a patient, I can unequivocally state that the grade realistically reflects a dramatic difference. I can say the same as a surgeon who works in these facilities. If I almost succumbed to a medical error when I fell at a hospital that had earned an A, think of the incidence of medical error in hospitals that score a C or worse.

The data alone is simply not enough.

And there is one other factor that requires government oversight of for-profit hospitals in the US, and that is the concept of budgeting.

A CEO of a for-profit hospital, for example, may craft a budget that projects profits of 30 million dollars. But as soon as it becomes clear that the hospital may only make profits of 10 million, they are suddenly "behind budget." When this occurs, people are laid off and corners are cut. In a traditional business, this may make sense. But remember, this is a hospital, not a Walmart. Reduced staff means patients will suffer. And all of this cutting happens not because the hospital is actually *losing* money, but simply because they won't make as much as they hoped.

Again, despite the fact that profiteering has no role in healthcare, our present system is allowing the dollar to win over the patient.

THE LACK OF national guidelines is a further problem in healthcare.

We have come to a point where every hospital is like a golf club: physicians must apply individually and present paperwork, and each hospital has different rules. In other words, hospitals function as fiefdoms. Imagine how frustrating (and illogical) it is when in one hospital I am told we must do something one way, while at another just a few miles away I am told to never do it that way. Because what is done in one hospital may not be done at another, it robs the healthcare system of efficiency—and this inefficiency permeates nearly all of medicine, including the licensing of physicians. When I needed a license years ago in Texas, I had to travel to Austin and physically present my original medical school diploma, despite its being framed, and take a 50-question jurisprudence test; whereas the state I was leaving, Iowa, required that I apply only by mail. Although the rules in Texas have softened considerably over the last 20 years, each state in the US has differing rules requiring physicians to pass various continuing medical education requirements. That means the licensing boards of New Jersey and Pennsylvania have different requirements for physicians, despite a river less than a few hundred feet wide separating the two.

A good way to illustrate this is to look at a chain like Burger King. They have thousands of stores in the US that reflect some degree of local characteristics, but the food is the same. Why? There are rules regarding how food is prepared so that customers can expect certain outcomes. In healthcare, however, where it has evolved over centuries within independent hospitals in differing states, there are no unifying processes. I realize this sounds like an argument for nationalizing healthcare, but I'm merely presenting in a logical fashion the issues we must consider. Everyone, regardless of economic standing, deserves the best possible care within standardized treatment algorithms. As a patient, I know I would have died had I been brought to some other hospitals in my region. If we had stricter national standards, this would rarely, if ever, be a statement I could truthfully make.

This makes absolutely no sense in our modern era. We have a unified defense system for our nation, why not a healthcare system?

PHYSICIAN DEBT AND DIMINISHING SALARIES FEED THE SYSTEM

One of the most attractive parts of being a physician, besides being a partner in the healing of patients, is the prospect of running your own practice, governed by the ethics, values, and standards you hold dear. In choosing your own staff, you set the tone for your office and for how patients are treated, from the front desk to the exam room to the surgical table. You have a great deal of control over how your practice is run.

But establishing a solo or even joint or group practice requires an enormous amount of capital. At the time of graduation, 86 percent of current medical school students carry over $190,000 in loans, and that number is growing every year, not to mention the thousands of dollars of interest that loan accumulates over time. Few can obtain yet another loan to open a practice, and when they can, the stress and strain of paying down this increasing debt only grows.

Why our country has not deemed reducing the cost of educating its physicians a national priority, thereby alleviating financial burden after graduation, makes little sense to me. Recently, a few medical schools have started to become tuition free, most notably NYU Medical School in 2019, funded by generous donors for a cool $450 million—but in the absence of that option, another great alternative would be to require that physicians serve in a public health service after graduation for a few years in exchange for a tuition-free education. Once their term was fulfilled, where they would no doubt hone valuable skills, they would be free to set up their own practices. Removing student loan burden from our future doctors would not only provide much-needed relief, but also open the door to scores of aspiring physicians who previously felt attending medical school was an impossible dream due to the crippling cost.

If I as a physician volunteer several weeks a year operating in Guatemala, why can't I do the same thing in Camden, New Jersey, or Detroit, Michigan, or any number of American cities where we could establish voluntary health services? Sadly, if I showed up at a charity hospital in a distant city such as Los Angeles, willing to volunteer my surgical skills for a few weeks, I would be laughed out of the building. That is a travesty.

As it stands presently, it's no surprise that fewer independent physicians exist due to the sheer financial expense and regulatory requirements to run a medical practice—not to mention that both the insurance companies and the government are actively ratcheting down physician reimbursement by linking full payment to specific and often bizarre metrics. As physicians become overwhelmed by this quickly changing system—and because it is so hard to survive on their own—they are now running into the open arms of the employed model, meaning employment by large for-profit medical groups. Although physicians are given a stable salary in that model, they lose autonomy and are subjugated to corporate shenanigans and to following the rules of the group, which means that patients are unwittingly subjected to even more cost-cutting. But because these doctors want and need to be paid, they tend to remain silent, even as they witness practices that are not in line with their Hippocratic Oath. Physicians are more likely to make their employer happy in order to continue receiving a paycheck than to speak up for patient care; when the employer of a physician is a hospital system, there is a definite conflict of interest. The physician is supposed to be an independent advocate for the patient, but how is that possible if the physician is paid by the hospital where the patient is being treated?

Tragically, this crisis has been hidden from the public, and the medical community has been loath to discuss it.

INCREASED MONEY-FOCUSED, NOT PATIENT-FOCUSED, PROCESSES

The last thing the population wants to hear is that physicians are under constant pressure to cut corners—but the truth is that's exactly what profit-driven healthcare dictates we do. This happens in any number of ways: shortening the patient's length of stay in a hospital so that the facility captures more money (recall my trach and PEG, then transfer to rehab); transferring a patient to a rehabilitation facility that is also owned by the same parent company, regardless of the overall quality; maximizing billing by capturing all diagnoses to generate reimbursements. All of it is unconscionable, and all of it hurts patients and doctors alike.

The electronic medical record (EMR) system holds physicians back from giving top-notch patient care too. These systems include designs that exploit the capturing of charges and track referrals, neither of which serves anything but the hospitals' bottom lines. In other words, EMRs basically serve as cash registers. The public is told that these EMRs improve safety, but the other half of the story is that they improve charge capture (also known as billing).

Here's an illustration of how this works.

During a patient visit, I am required to enter information into the hospital's EMR; in so doing, I am forced to link a diagnosis to help the hospital capture charges and bill. This is often akin to navigating a maze, which takes me away from vital patient interaction and has zero to do with patient safety. Even though I'm not employed by any of the hospitals where I attend, I must spend hours each day associating diagnoses with my orders and procedures to help the hospital capitalize its billing potential—and this is because hospitals have "released" (fired) the platoon of coders it previously employed to cull this data, instead transferring this task directly to physicians. It's an incredible waste of time to bang keys while the patient waits, hoping I pass a hard stop in the EMR program. I am no Luddite, but this is ridiculous.

To add further frustration, each hospital regularly changes and updates its EMR, such that if you attend several different places, it's nearly impossible to keep up with the varying systems. This is part of the for-profit strategy too: mastering one EMR chains physicians to a certain location, because learning a new system is completely overwhelming.

As I mentioned earlier, the EMR also tracks the referrals that are made, which adds yet another level of madness to an already faulty system. There was a time when doctors referred patients to whomever they felt was the best qualified specialist or colleague for the patient's situation, but now, unscrupulous administrators demand that their employed physicians refer only to doctors, regardless of skill, on the same financial team to try to keep costs down while maximizing revenue.

In sum, the ever-expanding EMRs take the doctor away from the patient. Physician dissatisfaction is at an all-time high because they are not doing what they went to medical school for: delivering patient care. This is another example of moral injury.

WHAT ARE WE TO DO?

I propose that, for a start, we look at our country's nonprofit charity hospitals as an appropriate model for all facilities.

Broadly speaking, there are two types of hospitals: 1) for-profit, and 2) nonprofit (also known as not-for-profit). But within the nonprofit rubric, there are those that make money but do not pay taxes (like many University facilities, for example), and then there are true charity hospitals (which are frequently run by a county or religious/service group).

As I mentioned at the beginning of this chapter, it's true that I've outlined ways I felt failed by the hospital after my trauma. But I also stated that it wasn't the *hospital* itself that failed me; it was the *system*.

The trauma hospital where I was treated is indeed geared, as a charity hospital, toward patient care, with its original mission being to fulfill a religious duty—a mission that was clear to everyone. I liken it to what Aristotle called Practical Reasoning: "A wise person does not use intuition alone but follows a path of logical thoughts to arrive at a rational solution." I viewed many employees of this hospital as imbued with this noble ethos, even as they were bound by old systems and protocols that didn't necessarily serve me well as a patient.

There were certainly staff members who stood out and truly served their mission: Maria, who carefully cleaned my ICU bay around Denise's visits; the ICU nurses who allowed Denise to stay slightly longer than permitted for visitation; the technicians who gently irrigated my trach; Jane the ICU nurse whose Irish lilt I will never forget as she treated me with tenderness. The individuals who initially started the hospital strove to ensure the mission was never abandoned. That mission of caring for anyone (patient or family member) in need was not lost on any employee. Indeed, this hospital is in an inner-city neighborhood where the staff see many injuries due to violence, yet they care for each person with equal attention.

Where the problems lie, and where I believe the slide away from patient-focused care was starting to occur in my healing experience, was where the goals of the facility focused more on the financial bottom line rather than my outcome as a patient. In order to remain viable, this hospital, like many in our country, was required to morph from pure charity to more nonprofit in its strategic financial management. Of course, a hospital must remain financially solvent and earn enough money to allow for the purchasing of new technology as well as the maintenance of the old, but perhaps hospital CEOs should instead refocus, like the founding members of our country's charity hospitals, on improving patient care while earning enough money to keep the doors open. But they need not be golden doors. In other words, just how much profit is enough for a charity or nonprofit hospital? This situation has become so dire, a nonprofit hospital in New Jersey was found to be essentially functioning so aggressively with regard to profiteering that the healthcare system that owned the facility was ordered to pay property taxes of $15.5 million over the next ten years for locations where making money was deemed the primary goal. The judge involved in the decision went on to say that nonprofit hospitals are arguably a legal fiction.[3] The fact that this did not make shockwaves in Washington, DC, speaks to the power of the healthcare industry.

While I certainly don't want to make assumptions about any person's intentions in the hospital in which I received care, I can say that the dismissive quality of some of the staff members, the over-sedation and restraining of patients, and the business-like way of some staff going about their shifts was a

---

[3] Meiksins, Mike. "Judge Terms Modern Nonprofit Hospitals a 'Legal Fiction.'" Nonprofit Quarterly. https://nonprofitquarterly.org/judge-terms-modern-nonprofit-hospitals-a-legal-fiction/ (accessed March 26, 2020).

reflection of precisely what might happen when a strictly charity model attempts to morph into capturing more revenue. The loving and humane treatment of patients starts to shrink in the face of monetary gain—which frequently translates to cutting corners, increasing staff ratios (fewer nurses for more patients), avoiding any possible litigation (from falls, patients pulling out tubes, etc., which increases with diminished staff), and a host of other issues I've brought to light in this book.

Having now been a patient in extremis, I would say there is an acute need to reinvigorate the true ethical mission of all our healthcare facilities throughout the nation. The calling of true service that was strictly enforced by the individuals who helped found the charity hospital that treated me must be instilled everywhere. Said another way, religious orders and service organizations do not have a monopoly on propagating this beneficent mission, as there are charity hospitals founded by certain county governments in our country that have risen to the occasion. Parkland in Dallas and Bellevue in New York City, both places I have worked, are to name but two. When leadership in these systems change, however, it can be easy for foundational principles to be forgotten and replaced. This is precisely what causes beloved institutions to spiral downward, not continue to grow upward.

And those antiquated systems and protocols I mentioned above?

My trauma hospital, with all the good intentions, was still mired in the use of certain procedures outdated in their construction and function—prolonged rigid endotracheal intubation, tracheostomy, and PEG, to name a few I experienced—simply because they are the only technologies available. This is true for all hospitals in the United States. Once again, we are utilizing technologies that have not been re-evaluated in decades. It would be like having only the option of using copper phone lines with four-pronged jacks in your newly purchased home; few people would tolerate that in the twenty-first century, yet nearly no one is challenging antiquated healthcare. As Elon Musk sets his sights on the cosmos, we need a similar-minded visionary championing a complete revamp of the tools we use in healthcare.

Healthcare workers cannot make procedures more physically tolerable with less scarring to a patient if the technology doesn't exist. Because of this, along with a shifted focus away from patient care toward a financial bottom line, even charity hospitals are suffering in their ability to provide the most care-centered patient experience. I had top-notch doctors and surgeons who saved my life, and nurses who sustained it, but they were still operating within a largely broken system.

This leads me to the final segment of this chapter.

ENSURING A CULTURE OF CARING

What my illness taught me is that all healthcare facilities, as well as the insurance industry, must have a culture of caring—and this culture *must* be the guiding mission no matter what the financial setup and at any cost. From the CEOs of for-profit hospitals to board members of the insurance industry, from the healthcare staff to the environmental staff, we must always put patient care above all else. As a society, we must re-evaluate the logic of the for-profit model in the healthcare industry, and we must ask if it is reasonable that many nonprofit hospitals are generating large amounts of profit that arguably should be redirected to delivery of healthcare. Bottom line: We need to have the charity model as our guiding force. These charity hospitals keep the doors open 24/7, provide outstanding quality care, and meet or exceed safety metrics, all while meeting financial requirements without gaming the system. The same must apply to the insurance and pharmaceutical industries. When this is the sincere mission, everything else becomes secondary. And when I say everything else, I mean all things that aren't primarily focused on helping patients heal and have the best quality of life.

This mindset can be achieved through a very simple exercise. For every element considered within our healthcare system, we must ask ourselves the following question:

Will [procedure, system, metric] help patients have the best healing experience?

For example:

Will investing in improving endotracheal tube engineering help patients have the best healing experience?

Will hitting our $30 million profit goal this year help patients have the best healing experience?

Will outlawing restraints and finding a better way to keep patients safe help them have the best healing experience?

Will letting go of 25 percent of the staff so we can report improved earnings help patients have the best healing experience?

Will funding low-interest, easy-to-obtain disability loans help patients have the best healing experience?

Will giving patients a cold, perfunctory description of a procedure help patients have the best healing experience?

Will giving patients a hand-held, compassionate description of a procedure help patients have the best healing experience?

Will minimizing coverage, or making it harder to reimburse, on higher-cost procedures help patients have the best healing experience?

Will eliminating unnecessary paperwork during a crisis situation help patients have the best healing experience?

Will setting the price of a drug at an affordable level for out-of-pocket purchase help the patient have the best healing experience?

I don't have to tell you how powerful it is to phrase all our interactions, our technologies, our medical training, and our goals in this way. Imagine a CEO, or the head of a hospital (whether nonprofit or for-profit), asking questions in this manner when making decisions. Same for the insurance or pharmaceutical industry. There's no gray area, and no room for abandoning the mission. If the question truly merits a no, we don't do it. If it merits a yes, we find a way—because nothing is more important than the mission: helping patients have the best healing experience.

Is solving the problems in the healthcare industry going to be this simple? No. But it's certainly a foundational start. When everything, *everything*, we do in medicine stems from what's best for patients, that's where we enter the space where we can't fail.

That's where we honor our Hippocratic Oath.

That's where our morality truly meets our mission.

After my fall from the roof, I was certainly close to death. I went into respiratory failure several times and required multiple emergent intubations. I am sad to say that at no time did I see a tunnel with white light, nor was I gifted any ethereal experiences by our Creator. But I do know this: I am the luckiest person in the world to have survived such a major ordeal and recover in a rapid fashion with essentially no significant long-term problems. I also believe that the biggest reason I endured what I did—in precisely the way I did—was to help start a long overdue discussion about our country's healthcare system.

I have no doubt that the team who cared for me saved my life. However, I also found it necessary to act as my own physician at times, when I was able, to expedite my recovery. Had I fully succumbed to my role of "patient" with all the bleak outcomes predicted for me by my doctors, who knows how long I might have taken to recover, if indeed I did recover completely.

I also can't help but give credit to the role of Fortuna—the Roman goddess of luck—in our daily lives. I've often asked myself: What if I fell at a different angle? What if my head had hit the concrete first? What if I had broken my femur and it pierced my skin and became infected? What if I'd been taken to a different hospital, the one my wife had initially requested? What if the ambulance driver hadn't insisted I be transported to the hospital that was more experienced in life-threatening injuries?

All these particular synchronicities added up to my having what feels like a fortunate trauma experience, one I can honestly say I've used to grow personally as well as professionally. Not only can I empathize with compassion as I work with patients who have terrible diagnoses and life-altering scars, but I can now also help them process the positive aspects of their struggle because I'm a living example. Helping people in this way gives me immense gratification, but there is so much more to be done.

I've outlined in this book much of what I believe this undertaking needs to encompass, and I certainly hope it will serve as a starting point. In one of the richest countries in the world, there is no excuse for the patient, and physician, suffering that occurs every day in our nation, all because not enough of us are making our voices heard in favor of the kind of patient care America can and should be providing—the kind America had before profit-based healthcare driven by massive corporations pushed preventative and holistic patient care to the wayside.

We have a big task before us to make the kind of sweeping changes I propose, but when healthcare workers and patients align, demanding both a logical and an advanced system of delivery geared solely toward preventing and curing illness, anything is possible.

Where there is life, there is hope.

addendum

◆

I wish to note that the publishing of this book in the midst of the COVID-19 pandemic is actually quite timely. The exact emotions the majority is now feeling—fear of death and the random nature of tragedy, disbelief, isolation, depression—are the same feelings addressed by this very book. The difference is that the emotions are currently global, not solely confined to patients in the ICU. Additionally, and certainly not coincidentally, this pandemic has exposed the very problems in healthcare explored in the pages you have just read.

WHAT YOU CAN DO

If you are a patient or family member:

As discussed, the healthcare team certainly has competing goals that indeed differ (even significantly) from you or your loved one. However, if you pose these questions daily in a non-confrontational manner, you can refocus everyone's attention to the most important issue: recovery. You can hold the healthcare team accountable, not necessarily for an ideal outcome, but rather for undertaking a transparent and concerted effort to attain the desired goal. These questions should be asked of the lead doctor, with the understanding that there is indeed someone coordinating and overseeing the team's efforts. You also should write the answers down and follow up with the team leader the next time rounds are performed.

Here are sample questions to help achieve the desired short-term outcome:

> *What is the most pressing primary goal today?*
>
> *Are there other primary goals we should know about?*
>
> *What measures are in place to achieve each of these goals?*
>
> *How is success measured for each of these goals?*
>
> *By what time will you know the outcome of each metric for success?*
>
> *How and when will that outcome be communicated to me?*
>
> *What if we don't achieve the anticipated outcome?*
>
> *How can I get in contact with a member of the medical team who has overseeing authority?*

By asking these questions politely and daily, you are holding the lead physician responsible for explaining the day's goal. As made clear, healing is a slow, step-by-step process. Not only should the short-term goals be elucidated (get off the ventilator, clear the infection), but long-term goals should be considered (transfer to a skilled nursing facility, wean off tracheostomy). This will require careful discussion with the lead physician on a frequent basis.

Here are sample questions regarding long-term goals:

What kind of help will I (or my loved one) need when I leave the hospital?

What will be the most challenging deficits for me (or my loved one)?

What resources will I (or my loved one) need after discharge?

How do I (or my loved one) access these resources?

To where will I (or my loved one) be discharged?

How can someone I trust inspect the facility where I (or my loved one) will be transferred prior to arrival?

Do you or anyone on the healthcare team have a financial interest in the facility where I (or my loved one) will be transferred?

Recommendations for family members:

- Illness is traumatic, and some degree of familial conflict is inevitable regardless of how much love is present. This is only natural, but hopefully, it will be more minor than major. Remember that it is the patient who must remain first and foremost the center of attention. This can be exhausting; nevertheless, all actions must be geared toward helping the patient return to as normal as possible, regardless of how you feel personally. Always act in the best interest of the patient—not what you *think* is in his or her best interest but rather what you think the patient would *want*.

- If conflict arises, recognize it. Ask for forgiveness, which requires recognition of the reciprocity of hurt. And be aware that for an apology to be successful, you must be concerned solely about the hurt you caused the *patient*, not the hurt that *you* may feel. In other words, admit your mistakes and enumerate these actions as harmful, but do not defend or justify them. In defining how your actions caused strife, you take true ownership and are mindful of what your specific actions caused. Be patient but persistent in winning back trust.

If you are a healthcare worker:

Illness is a terrifying event that everyone is likely to experience at some time in his or her life.

- Never forget the vulnerability patients and their families feel. Although people say to treat a patient as you would want to be treated, this is not wholly accurate. Some people like the hard truth, whereas others may be better served with supportive caring. It is your job as a physician or nurse to discern and try to work with a patient and his or her family in the best way that works for *them*, not *you*. To successfully achieve this, you must make the time to dedicate yourself to and navigate this critical process. Treat the patient as if they are indeed *family*. That means you may treat one patient somewhat differently than another, just like you may handle your aunt and your grandmother in a different fashion. But all your interactions with family are based on love. This should always be reflected.

- Never forget your Hippocratic Oath.

- Being overworked or overburdened will never lead to a successful outcome when interacting with a patient. Rushing or having a curt temper is a formula for failure. This means that you must know accurately how long rounds or clinic visits will take. You must not allow yourself to be over-scheduled. If you are, you must apologize for this and put measures in place preventing it from becoming a frequent occurrence. Generally, you should run on time and account for delays with appropriate scheduling. By definition, emergencies occur and rushed encounters will happen. These must be infrequent; however, if you find yourself without enough time to be the physician you wish more often than not, you must carefully analyze your scheduling and your goals.

- Always acknowledge the patient. Recognize the fear and pain he or she is experiencing. Ask the patient if you are meeting his or her expectations. Ask what you can do better. Synthesize and learn from the answer.

- Never forget the family members of your patient. Recognize them and thank them for their help.

Acknowledge their constant vigil. Thank them for their love. Encourage their prayer.

- If you are employed, investigate mechanisms available to identify lapses in patient safety while not risking your job. Always be mindful of your tone but remain cognizant that simply identifying safety issues can make you a problem in the eyes of your employer. If that is the case, consider finding employment in a healthcare system that truly places the patient first. Remember that you alone cannot change a broken system, or fight a system as a whistleblower when they have a much deeper pocket.

RESOURCES

There are several independent websites that measure and compare facilities, and these metrics are critical. Things such as surgical site infections, patient falls, or meaningful communication are measured and tracked. On the other hand, reviews left by patients on Google or Yelp should be eschewed. Sadly, people die in hospitals because some illness is simply too big to cure. As a result, some reviews on public websites are inaccurate or vindictive.

Search and compare some of your favorite local hospitals—and don't be surprised if you're shocked:

www.medicare.gov/hospitalcompare
www.leapfroggroup.org/compare-hospitals

Daily, at least 1 in 31 patients in hospitals suffer a hospital-acquired infection. Explore this website to become informed about why it's important to advocate for patients:

www.cdc.gov/hai/data/index.html

Fear and conflict during illness is inevitable. Having a religious framework is helpful for some, and turning toward clergy can indeed provide deep solace. For others, a philosophical outlook is more valuable. For those who have an interest in Stoic philosophy as I do, this website provides daily pithy insights:

www.dailystoic.com

If conflict arises between family members, consider step 8 of the 12-step Program of Alcoholics Anonymous. Although this may seem rash, this step successfully helps guide people who are lost in the process of asking forgiveness from those whom they have transgressed. For more information regarding this step:

www.aa.org/assets/en_US/en_step8.pdf

Although PICS (or, as I suggest it become renamed, PPICS) and PTSD are well known consequences of treating severe illness, most healthcare facilities simply ignore these significant issues. The Critical Illness, Brain Dysfunction, and Survivorship (CIBS) Center at Vanderbilt University does an outstanding job of enumerating symptoms, causes, and treatments. You can learn more about this and encourage local ICUs to follow these protocols:

www.ICUdelirium.org

Whether you are a healthcare worker or a patient, this website shines a bright light on our dysfunctional healthcare system. It is simultaneously shocking and humorous:

www.zdoggmd.com

ACKNOWLEDGMENTS

An endeavor such as this requires recognition of all those who made it possible behind the scenes. I think the answer is obvious when it is a near-death experience.

First and foremost are those anonymous individuals who were simply performing their jobs on December 22, 2018, and thereafter: To the first-aid squad members, interns, residents, nurses, physicians, therapists, and housekeeping staff, I am so grateful.

To my sincere friends who have been there for my recovery and afterwards, I am grateful.

And most importantly, to my spouse, my ultimate life partner: Words are insufficient. I recall resting in bed while in rehab and describing to you how our marriage was no accident, although our meeting certainly was (or maybe it was indeed Fortuna raising her head once again?). I compared how my waiting for you was like a sniper, sitting in camouflaged cover looking through a scope, patiently waiting to calmly pull the trigger on the one proper target. I have never, not once, regretted my actions.

This would never have been possible but for the folks at Miles Trevor Press.

I am especially grateful to Stacey Aaronson. Her hard work, patience, expertise, and insight as an editor are greatly appreciated.

ABOUT THE AUTHOR

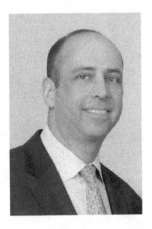

ROSS I.S. ZBAR, MD, FACS, is a reconstructive plastic surgeon in solo private practice located in northern New Jersey. Following his graduation magna cum laude in biology from Harvard College, he earned his MD at Yale University School of Medicine and completed his internship in general surgery at Lenox Hill Hospital in New York City. He trained in Otolaryngology – Head and Neck Surgery at the University of Iowa Hospitals and Clinics as well as Plastic Surgery at the University of Texas Southwestern Medical Center at Dallas. He holds board certification in both surgical specialties and undertook further training in craniofacial surgery as the first Jerome P. Webster fellow. As a scientific author, he is often published and cited in peer-reviewed journals. *Floating Feathers* is his initial foray into non-scientific literature.